GROW WITH SYMPATHY, EMPATHY, & COMPASSION

PROVIDE GENUINE SUPPORT AND WITNESS PROFOUND RECOVERY

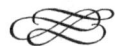

KIANNAH FROST

© 2020 by Kiannah Frost

All rights reserved. The content contained within this book may not be reproduced, duplicated or transmitted without direct written permission from the author or the publisher.

Under no circumstances will any blame or legal responsibility be held against the publisher, or author, for any damages, reparation, or monetary loss due to the information contained within this book, either directly or indirectly.

Legal Notice:

This book is copyright protected. It is only for personal use. You cannot amend, distribute, sell, use, quote or paraphrase any part, or the content within this book, without the consent of the author or publisher.

Disclaimer Notice:

Please note the information contained within this document is for educational and entertainment purposes only. All effort has been executed to present accurate, up to date, reliable, complete information. No warranties of any kind are declared or implied. Readers acknowledge that the author is not engaged in the rendering of legal, financial, medical or professional advice. The content within this book has been derived from various sources. Please consult a licensed professional before attempting any techniques outlined in this book.

By reading this document, the reader agrees that under no circumstances is the author responsible for any losses, direct or indirect, that are incurred as a result of the use of the information contained within this document, including, but not limited to, errors, omissions, or inaccuracies.

CONTENTS

Dear Reader   vii
Introduction: Reconnect With Others   ix

Part I
WHAT IS SYMPATHY?

The Concept of Sympathy	3
The Two Fundamental Types of Sympathy	5
What is Sympathy Related To?	8
What Causes Feelings of Sympathy?	12

Part II
THE BENEFITS OF SYMPATHY AND HOW TO USE IT

7 Reasons to Live with Sympathy	17
Thoughts to Keep in Mind When Showing Sympathy	22
Three Ways of Showing Sympathy to Others	27

Part III
WHEN SYMPATHY GOES WRONG

What To Avoid When Showing Sympathy to Others	35
Situations Where You May Not Want To Show Sympathy	38
Let Your Walls Down, But Learn to Put Them Back Up	41

Part IV
WHAT IS EMPATHY?

The Three Main Types of Empathy	47
How Does Empathy Differ from Sympathy?	51
The Science Behind Empathy	53

Part V
THE BENEFITS OF EMPATHY AND HOW TO BE MORE EMPATHETIC

The Benefits of Empathy to Yourself and Others	59
Becoming a More Empathetic Individual	63
Expressing Your Empathy to Others	67

Part VI
WHEN EMPATHY WORKS AGAINST YOU

What Happens When You Misuse Empathy?	75
Important Things to Keep in Mind with Showing Empathy to Others	77
Situations Where You Should Avoid Using Empathy	80

Part VII
WHAT IS COMPASSION?

Defining Compassion	85
How Compassion Differs from Sympathy and Empathy	88
The Science Behind Compassion	93

Part VIII
THE BENEFITS OF COMPASSION AND HOW TO LEAD A MORE COMPASSIONATE LIFE

What are the Benefits of Being Compassionate?	101
When Should Compassion be Used?	105
How To Lead a More Compassionate Life	107
Compassion in Daily Life	112

Part IX
THE DOWNSIDE OF COMPASSION

Can Compassion Be a Weakness?	119
How Does Compassion Become Painful?	122
When Compassion Doesn't Work	125
Knowing When the Situation Requires Compassion	127

Part X
USING SYMPATHY, EMPATHY, AND
COMPASSION IN YOUR LIFE

Scenario 1: Showing Sympathy to Ease the Pain of Loss	133
Scenario 2: Empathizing to Show Support	135
Scenario 3: Empathizing to Spread Happiness	137
Scenario 4: A Challenging Way to Show Compassion	139
Thank You For Reading	143
Conclusion: Making Positive Changes in Your Life	144
About the Author	147
References	149

Dear Reader,

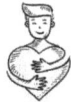 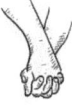 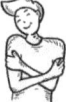

Thank you so much for purchasing this book. I hope that you will find valuable information that you can use to enrich your life and grow with sympathy, empathy, and compassion. I would like to offer you free early access and excerpts of my next book—it's super exciting, and I can't wait to share it with you all. You can sign up to get involved using the link below or by scanning the QR code.

kiafrost.com/earlyreader

— KIA

INTRODUCTION: RECONNECT WITH OTHERS

We are all familiar with the words: sympathy, empathy, and compassion.

But do you know what these words mean? Do you truly know how to be sympathetic, empathetic, and compassionate? And did you know that these are some of the most powerful tools that you can use to make a positive change in someone's life? Even your own!

While many people use these terms—and even interchangeably—many don't know the difference between them. Also, they may not know how to use these beautiful tools to help themselves and others around them. It's time to learn what these terms mean and how they can cause a ripple of positive effects in your life.

You picked up the perfect book as this aims to provide you with concrete definitions of sympathy, empathy, and compassion. Understanding what these terms truly mean will enlighten you so that you can use them appropriately. Here, you will also be learning how to apply these tools to different situations in your life and different contexts. I even share examples to make it easier for you to understand everything better. Of course, as with any other tools or virtues, these three have their dark sides. And I will also help you learn where each of these can go wrong and how to avoid such situations.

In the past, I believed that I was a genuinely sympathetic, empathetic, and compassionate person. Raised by my kind mother, I learned about these feelings from a young age. Whenever I would meet someone experiencing grief, I would sympathize with them. Whenever I would run into someone experiencing hardships, I would empathize with them. Whenever I would communicate with someone experiencing an awkward situation, I would feel compassion for them. But that's it. I would feel these things, but I wouldn't go beyond those feelings.

That is until I tried learning more about sympathy, empathy, and compassion.

I have always been a life-long learner of everything related to psychology. Even before I studied psychology, I was interested in learning more about human behavior and what makes us tick. In particular, I have tried to learn everything that I can about emotional intelligence and its importance in our lives. Through thousands of hours of research and real-life applications, I can confidently say that I have gained profound knowledge of the concepts of sympathy, empathy, and compassion. I have seen how these tools have made a positive impact on the lives of those close to me. And though this book, you can grow with sympathy, empathy, and compassion too.

One of the most important benefits you will be able to take from this book is that you will understand the meaning of each of these valuable tools properly. Because of this, you will be able to communicate more effectively with the people around you and know what to do when things start turning sour. You can use these tools to

INTRODUCTION: RECONNECT WITH OTHERS

improve your existing relationships, create new connections, and grow yourself in ways you never even thought were possible.

Right now, I want to make a promise to you. If you apply everything you learn from this book in the real world, you will be able to uplift those around you. In doing this, you will also uplift yourself, thus, allowing you to live a more fulfilled life. Being able to build better connections with other people is just the beginning. The things you are about to learn will also enable you to handle tough conversations to ignite your personal growth.

With all of these beautiful things that can potentially happen in your life, why wait any longer? There's no better time than the present to start skilling up and improving yourself. The good news is that you have already taken the all-important first step by purchasing this book. Now, it's time for you to start learning how to apply knowledge about sympathy, empathy, and compassion to transform the lives of the people around you and your own in the process. You already have the key to unlocking the wealth of knowledge in your hand. Now all you have to do is keep turning the pages.

Each chapter of this book is essential for you to understand, build, and use the tools you need to work with other people more effectively and help yourself grow. As you read this book, take notes, highlight phrases that resonate with you, and write down your ideas in a notebook or on post-it notes. Then, stick these notes all-around your room to keep you motivated. Do what you think is best to make this learning experience, one that will stick with you for the rest of your life. And with this last piece of valuable advice, let's begin your journey!

PART I
WHAT IS SYMPATHY?

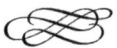

Sympathy is a feeling you get when you see unfortunate things happening to the people around you. When you sympathize with someone, you feel bad for them because of the difficulties they are experiencing. Often, you would feel the most sympathy towards someone who has lost someone close to them because of death. In this case, you will often hear other people say, "I feel for them" or "I sympathize with them." This feeling is the most basic explanation of sympathy. But as a concept and as a tool for changing your life, there's much more to it.

As you begin to improve your understanding of sympathy, you will learn that it relates to empathy and compassion. These virtues are similar as well, and learning how to use them correctly—while knowing when you shouldn't use them—is key to making a change in your life. The ability to feel sympathy for other people is an essential part of being human. Sympathy can also be an invisible force that compels you to reach out to others to offer assistance.

The main thing that differentiates sympathy from empathy and compassion is that with sympathy, you can feel bad for other people even if you have never experienced their situation, or you are not experiencing the same feelings as them. At this point, since it is the beginning of the book, you may be feeling a bit confused, and that's all right. Throughout this book, we will be discussing the differences between these three terms. By the end, you will be able to understand—and apply—these tools in the best possible way.

THE CONCEPT OF SYMPATHY

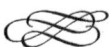

The concept of sympathy is quite simple. Sympathy means to feel sorry for a person that is experiencing hurt or pain. When you feel sympathy, you still maintain some level of emotional distance with the person. You may not feel the same emotions as the other person. Instead, you would think that it's sad for the person to experience what they're feeling. In some cases, especially when your feelings of sympathy are powerful, you can instead feel pity for the person. However, try to be careful with how you express this as most people don't appreciate being the object of pity.

Pity is an emotion that may stem from sympathy. But doesn't have the same positive connotation. Those who feel pity tend to belittle and dehumanize the person who is experiencing a bad situation. In turn, this might cause offense to them, especially if they don't want other people to pity them. On the other hand, when you feel sympathy for the person, you may feel bad for them, but you won't make them feel any worse about their situation.

Sympathy comes from the Greek words "syn"—

meaning together—and "pathos"—meaning feeling. It refers to your ability to perceive, understand, and react to the pain, need, or distress of others. The source of sympathy is a shift in perspective. Instead of seeing things from your perspective, you will see them through the view of the person or persons in need. This perspective shift happens because our minds, as human beings, are similar in how they work and how they feel.

Sympathy evolved in human beings, along with the development of our social intelligence. The word itself refers to a wide range of behaviors along with the cognitive skills associated with them. According to different theories, sympathetic emotions exist because of reciprocal altruism. Our desire to build mutually beneficial relationships drives our emotions. In turn, we can understand how other people feel, to either avoid danger or ensure positive outcomes.

The term sympathy is often used interchangeably with empathy. While these are both feelings that we can experience, their meanings and origins are different. When you feel sympathetic, you won't necessarily share the same feelings as the person experiencing something for themselves. As a concept, sympathy can also refer to how you understand the reasons and thinking of another person. So, when they encounter challenges, you may end up feeling bad for them.

Used correctly, this would lead you to try and help the other person. While this is an appropriate reaction, there are proper and improper ways to offer help. Also, learning when to learn when expressing sympathy or when it's better for you to keep your thoughts to yourself is critical. That way, you can improve your relationships with other people and make more positive connections with them no matter how difficult things get for you or those around you.

THE TWO FUNDAMENTAL TYPES OF SYMPATHY

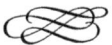

In some ways, sympathy can be a mutual understanding that comes from a similarity of feeling. When you understand another person's feelings, this means that you are sympathizing with them. And once you act on these feelings, sympathy becomes a powerful tool for change. The more genuine your sympathy is towards another person, the more powerful its impact is.

While sympathy comes easily for some people, others have to work on developing it. There are different types of sympathy and knowing them enables you to determine whether sympathy is already a part of who you are, or if it is an area for improvement. Let's take a look at the two types of sympathy and what they mean:

1. INNATE SYMPATHY

In 2006, a group of researchers from Switzerland conducted a study about sympathy in children (Malti et al., 2009). Through this study, they wanted to find out whether the sympathy that children show is for their benefit or if it was an innate aspect of their development. The researchers of this study concluded that sympathy is, in fact, a natural part of development. Even without the guidance of parents, children can develop both sympathy and empathy as they grow up. Also, the researchers discovered that girls tend to be more prosocial, morally motivated, and sympathetic compared to boys.

This study is critical, as it proves that we all have the potential to show sympathy. It is part of who we are, and thus, it is innate. As you were growing up, sympathy was already a part of you. But if you didn't use it or you never really felt it, it might have been buried deep within you. Despite this, you can still learn to be sympathetic—and this is the other type of sympathy you can have.

2. LEARNED SYMPATHY

Even children who are as young as 1-year-old can show sympathy towards other people. For instance, if a 1-year-old baby cries because they hear another baby crying, this may show sympathy. Or if a 1-year old gives one of their toys to another child without being asked for it, they might be feeling bad for the other child. These simple acts show primary sympathetic responses that come from their innate ability to feel sympathy.

Conversely, some aren't used to expressing their sympathy. These children may grow up without learning how to use or express this feeling. For instance, a child may grow up with parents who are too busy to spend time with them. As this child grows and develops, their interactions revolve around babysitters, children in daycare centers, and other adults who aren't their parents. Since these adults aren't the parents of the child, they might not be as invested in the child's growth and development. Therefore, they may not take the time to show the child how to express their feelings appropriately—and one such feeling is sympathy.

When that child grows up, they might not know how to show sympathy. Fortunately, both children and adults can learn how to sympathize. And the more they practice or use this, the better they get at it.

WHETHER INNATE OR LEARNED, sympathy remains to be a valuable and useful tool. As long as you use sympathy to affect change, it doesn't matter what type you have. The important thing is to know how to use it in the best and most appropriate ways.

WHAT IS SYMPATHY RELATED TO?

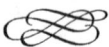

Sympathy is a feeling, a virtue, and a tool you can use to initiate the start of beautiful new things in your life. When you can feel sympathy, it means that you also can understand what other people are feeling. Through sympathy, you can either imagine or understand why a person is feeling sad, anxious, or distressed about their situation. While you may not share the other person's feelings, you can understand them. Thus, you can provide comfort as needed.

The more you understand sympathy, the more you will realize how much it is related and different to pity, empathy, and compassion. Sympathy is also related to your Emotional Quotient (EQ) as those who can show sympathy appropriately have a higher Emotional Quotient. Sympathy, empathy, and compassion are hallmark traits of people with a high EQ. People with high EQ can recognize emotions, understand the effects of these emotions, and use the information they have learned from that understanding to guide thoughts and behaviors.

Although many people consider sympathy as a basic

human trait, many people don't know how to use it properly. When this happens, it hinders your ability to connect more profoundly with other people, even with those whom you already know. Also, not knowing how to sympathize with other people properly can lead to hurting those you love instead of helping or healing them. Without genuine sympathy, you may not be able to distance yourself from the emotions felt by those going through tough times. And this is where things can go wrong.

Learning the difference between sympathy and empathy (and compassion) is fundamental for personal growth. While this isn't such an easy task since these concepts are very similar to each other, you may understand them more once you begin to apply them in your life. Sympathy is where you understand what another person is feeling from a distance. On the other hand, empathy is where you would experience the same feelings as the person who is undergoing pain, stress, and other emotions. To help you understand what these terms mean, let me share an example with you.

For instance, one of your friend's mothers has passed away. When you sympathize with your friend, you will try to understand and recognize the feelings your friend is having, such as sadness, pain, or even anger. But when you empathize with your friend, you would feel the same emotions as them. In turn, the reactions you would have to the sympathy or empathy you felt would differ as well.

When you sympathize, you can send a sympathy note, offer kind words, and make some simple but meaningful gestures to show support. While you aren't feeling your friend's pain, you understand that they are undergoing something difficult. Thus, you want them to know that you're aware of what they are feeling. For many people, this feels natural to do. Try to imagine how difficult it would be for you to experience the same emotions as your friend, who has just lost their mother. As your friend grieves, so will you. And this is what makes empathy much more challenging to experience.

Another term that is closely related to sympathy—and empathy—is compassion. Compassion is when you would feel sincere sympathy for the pain or sorrow of another person. Because of this, you may have a strong compulsion to do something about easing their pain. Compassion involves sympathy but expects action beyond understanding. For instance, if you have a friend who just gave birth, and they are struggling with everything they have to deal with, you can show compassion by helping out with a few of their chores. Although you won't gain anything from helping out, you would still do it to make your friend's challenges a little bit easier.

Finally, sympathy is also related to pity, as I mentioned earlier. Although this isn't one of the tools that can help improve your life, knowing what pity is can help you be more careful when you feel or experience it. When you feel pity, you may have a kind (and condescending) feeling of sorrow for another person brought about by that person's situation. Often, when you feel pity for someone, you would tend to feel sorry for them. That is why I won't be encouraging you to pity others as much as sympathy, empathy, or compassion.

Sympathy is also known as "community of feeling" or "fellow feeling." You experience sympathy when you feel concerned, or you care for another person because you understand their situation and what they're feeling. When you compare sympathy to pity, the former comes with deeper personal engagement and a more authentic sense of concern. Because of this, people who are undergoing stressful situations are more accepting of sympathy than

GROW WITH SYMPATHY, EMPATHY, & COMPASSION

they are of pity. When you sympathize with someone, they would feel good about it. But when you take pity on them, they might resent you for it.

Understanding the virtues and tools that are related to sympathy is essential as it enables you to comprehend what it means entirely. And now that you know what sympathy is related to, you can focus on the causes and how to use it in the best way possible.

WHAT CAUSES FEELINGS OF SYMPATHY?

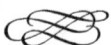

Sympathy is a feeling that doesn't just come out of thin air. For you to experience sympathy for another person, several things happen, including:

- A person experiences a problematic situation or could be in some need.
- You recognize and understand the pain or stress that this person feels. It's even more effective if you're close to or care about them.
- You aren't distracted by anything as this can hinder your ability to feel sympathetic towards them.

When you meet all of these conditions, you would feel sympathy for another person. The level of sympathy that you feel would depend on the level of pain or need that you perceive. For instance, you may not feel as sympathetic towards someone who falls and scrapes their elbow compared to someone who falls and fractures their wrist.

GROW WITH SYMPATHY, EMPATHY, & COMPASSION

Naturally, the direr the situation, the more sympathetic you would feel towards them.

As you can imagine, sympathy is a very subjective feeling. In some cases, you might even feel more sympathetic towards a person who is in a situation you have already experienced. The causes and levels of your sympathetic feelings may also depend on your perception, social connection, and even mood. For instance, if your friend loses money on an investment, you may feel very sympathetic towards them if you had experienced the same situation in the past. Conversely, if you hear about a situation that you haven't experienced yet, the level of sympathy you experience may not be as intense.

Your current state of mind can also impact the way that you feel and perceive sympathy. For example, negative emotions of your own can become distractions. While you are dealing with your problems, you may not be able to focus on the difficulties of others. Thus, you may not feel sympathetic towards them. Another example is that you could feel extremely positive because you feel confident as you have just finished your last exam. However, one of your friends who still has not completed their final exam may still be quite stressed and not feel the same positive energy as you.

PART II
THE BENEFITS OF SYMPATHY AND HOW TO USE IT

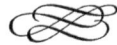

By now, you should already have a better understanding of sympathy. At its very core, sympathy is the ability to understand a person's situation and the feelings that they are experiencing. When you sympathize with them, you don't have to share the same feelings. You feel bad for them, and because of this, you can express your sympathy in suitable ways.

But what if you don't know anyone who has experienced pain, discomfort, or grief in their life?

Strange as this may seem, some people are lucky enough to go through life without experiencing deep pain or sadness. Of course, this doesn't mean that their lives are better than mine, yours or anyone else's. More likely, they experience pain, but they are just more resilient. Instead of telling other people about the troubles they are going through, they deal with their problems and move on. And if most of those around you are like this, you might not have much experience with feeling or expressing sympathy.

Still, at some point, there will come a time when someone in your life will lean on you for support. And when this happens, you should be ready. Now that you understand what sympathy is, it's time to learn what sympathy can bring to your life and how you can use it properly.

7 REASONS TO LIVE WITH SYMPATHY

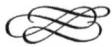

$\mathcal{S}$ympathy is a special feeling as it enables you to care for another person and want things to become better for them. Unlike empathy, you don't feel the same emotions. Instead, you feel care, concern, and sometimes, even a compulsion to help—and this leads to compassion. Through sympathy, you feel strongly about the situation of another person in a positive way. When you think about it, sympathy feels good because it causes you to care more about the people you love the most. And the more you care, the stronger your connections with others become. Of course, this good feeling isn't the only benefit of sympathy. Let's take a look at the other positive things that you can experience through sympathy:

- **It improves your social life.**

The ability to sympathize with other people by understanding the emotions they feel when faced with difficult situations plays a vital role in your social life. Understanding the perils of others and sympathizing with them opens your eyes to other perspectives and makes you more accepting of other people. Instead of judging others because of how they feel or how they react, you would, instead, choose to sympathize with them and even try to help them deal with their challenges.

When other people see that you are genuinely sympathetic, they will know that they can turn to you when they are in need. Even if you don't do anything concrete to help them out, the mere fact that you are listening to them and you genuinely care for them says a lot about who you are as a person. Naturally, when others see you this way, they may feel a safer connection with you.

- **It helps to expand your support system.**

As human beings, it is our nature to be social creatures, and we tend to depend on other people to confirm our own beliefs. When someone is in an unfortunate situation and feel like they cannot get out of it, they may need support. You may be one of those people who provides support, and if so, this will help your support system grow. When you are there for others in their times of need, they will not hesitate to show you the same sympathy and care when you are the one who needs help. We all need a robust support system. Fortunately, sympathy can help with this too.

- **It strengthens your emotions and your morality.**

You can also consider sympathy as a form of emotional and moral support. When you show sympathy to others, you are also showing them that they matter to you. Even though their difficult situation may negatively impact their life, they know that they don't have to go through it alone. Even if they don't accept your help or they think they may be better off without it, at least you have offered your support. Also, make sure that you are available if they reach out to you. Doing good deeds for others helps strengthen your moral compass as it reinforces positive behaviors.

- **It's something you can use no matter where you are and who you are with.**

No matter where you are and whom you're with, you can sympathize with others to help them feel better. Sympathy is an abstract concept, but it does have concrete effects like providing comfort, conveying concern, and improving the wellness of others. As long as you know how to express genuine sympathy, you can use it to enrich your life and the lives of those around you. Be wary, though—not everyone enjoys being the subject of sympathy. Make sure that it is appropriate and genuine so that you do not offend the people you are trying to support.

- **It helps you learn how to ask for help when you find yourself facing challenges.**

Many people struggle to reach out to others to ask for help. This challenge can come from differences in culture and social norms. Some people find it easy to share and reach out when they need help, whereas some people prefer to bottle up their emotions. The more you practice expressing sympathy, the more you will understand what it truly means. And when you find yourself in a situation where you're the one in need, you won't hesitate to ask for help. You're more likely to be comfortable asking for help from others. Usually, these people would be part of your support system—the one you've built by showing genuine sympathy.

- **It makes you more attractive to others.**

Even if you're not looking for a lifelong partner (or you've already found one), being more sympathetic can make you more attractive. It makes much sense when you think about it because when you express sympathy, it shows your softer, more emotional side. People are generally attracted to qualities of kindness, forgiveness, and love (I know that I am), and practicing sympathy can help improve these desirable qualities.

Knowing how to use sympathy can also help if you become a parent (or if you're already a parent). Studies have shown that sympathetic parents have the potential to raise children who are more caring and resilient.

- **It is one of our strongest instincts.**

Finally, it's also important to note that sympathy is a basic human instinct—and it is one of the most powerful. As mentioned in the previous chapter, sympathy is an innate character quality that develops over time. As we develop our ability to express genuine sympathy, the more natural it becomes. And when you're able to use sympathy in the best way, you can enjoy all the other benefits I've listed here.

You can think of it as a never-ending positive loop. The more you use sympathy, the more beneficial it becomes. And the more benefits you experience, the more you feel

GROW WITH SYMPATHY, EMPATHY, & COMPASSION

motivated to use it to change the lives of others (and yourself) for the better.

As YOU CAN TELL, there are many benefits of showing sympathy to others in need. Whether you're growing yourself or helping others (ideally both simultaneously), learning the skills to execute genuine sympathy is critical. This next section outlines the most important things to keep in mind when expressing sympathy.

THOUGHTS TO KEEP IN MIND WHEN SHOWING SYMPATHY

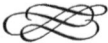

It's the perfect time for you to learn about some of the things that I keep in mind when using sympathy. It doesn't matter how good we think we are at showing sympathy to others or how much experience we have at being sympathetic. There are a few critical things that I always try to remember. By no means is this an exhaustive list, but it's an excellent starting point to living with more genuine sympathy:

- **Try to relate with others appropriately.**

Whether you have experienced the same situation as another person or they are going through something you have no experience with, you should work to understand them. It's easy to fall into the trap of making the situation about you, and this is something you should try and consciously avoid. If you were able to get over the same issue in the past, it doesn't mean that other people will be able to bounce back as quickly or as easily as you. It's better to listen to those in pain or need as this will help you better understand the situation that they are in and the feelings that they have.

After listening to a person and gaining a good understanding of their feelings, it's time for you to find the best way to relate with that person. You may share words of sympathy then ask how you can help. If you feel like the person isn't ready to accept help yet, assure them that you are there to provide whatever support they need. Relating to another person means that you can offer advice appropriately. And when you can do this, it shows that your sympathy is genuine and profound.

- **Try not to bring issues of faith to the conversation.**

If you're a person of faith, this may help you as you assist someone who is going through a difficult time. Just remember that not all people may rely on faith as you do. For instance, before giving advice, try to take a moment to reflect on their perspective and beliefs.

Unless you know for a fact that the person relies strongly on faith as much as you, it might not sit well with them. In some cases, the person might get offended by your actions. Therefore, it's best to steer clear of issues of faith when you're trying to express your sympathy.

- **Assure the other person that they are in your thoughts.**

Providing assurance is an excellent step to take if you notice that the person you are feeling sympathetic towards isn't ready to talk about or deal with their issues. In some cases, people may not want to talk about their situation.

And in some cases, they may be willing to speak, but not to you. Try not to take it personally!

Let them know that they can rely on you for support whenever they are ready to ask for it. This gesture provides comfort to the person and could make them feel better. Of course, when the time comes that they do call on you for help, make sure that you will deliver. Otherwise, they might see you as someone who says good things but never follows through.

- **Be generous, within reason.**

Often, when people experience difficult times in their lives, they may feel overwhelmed with emotion. When this happens, their lives may come to a halt as they try to understand what happened, react to the situation, and try to process their emotions. And as they try to keep everything together, they may not think about asking for help.

During these times, try to be proactive and overly generous without overstepping boundaries. After you express sympathy, you can also ask them if there is anything you can do to help. However, try not to force it. If they politely decline, follow-up by telling them that they can always reach out to you when they need to. If they ask you what you want to do to help, try to think of practical ways, such as offering to help with chores at home, driving your friend around town, or providing meals or snacks.

Often, people who are in difficult situations end up neglecting the things they would usually do in their lives. Providing the opportunity for a helping hand makes your sympathetic gestures more appropriate and useful.

- **Try not to force the person to deal with their problem right away.**

GROW WITH SYMPATHY, EMPATHY, & COMPASSION

It's important to give others personal space when they are facing challenges. Imagine how you would feel if you experienced something painful, and those around you keep telling you to get over it or move on. You might end up resenting them or feeling even worse about your situation.

There is no need for you to rush a person to feel better, nor is there a need to force them to deal with their situation. Always remember that we all have our ways of grieving and coping with problems and stress. Even if something seems minor to you, the other person might see the same situation as overwhelming. So try and give them space and allow them to cope. And when they are ready, that's when you can help out.

- **Keep in touch with the people in your life.**

It's best to know what's going on in people's lives before reaching out to them if you want to show genuine sympathy. To do this, you may want to keep in touch with them. Imagine, for example, how bad you would feel if you heard about one of your closest friends who experienced a death in the family over a month ago.

Even if you sympathize with them, the timing and impact of your sympathy wouldn't be as powerful as it could have been if you heard the news right after it happened. You don't have to overcommunicate with the people in your life if you choose not to, but keeping in touch with them is valuable. This communication enables you to show and use genuine sympathy when the need arises.

If you keep these six simple pointers in the back of your

mind, the next time you express sympathy towards others might be more appropriate and impactful. Maybe you will see profound recovery, or at the minimum, you will grow with sympathy. In this next chapter, we explore the three ways of showing your sympathy to others.

THREE WAYS OF SHOWING SYMPATHY TO OTHERS

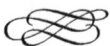

*D*epending on the situation, there are appropriate and inappropriate ways of showing sympathy to others. You may feel comfortable using your words. Alternatively, a non-verbal approach may be suited better for the person you are supporting. Either way, you should try and continue to show sympathy over time. I have emphasized how sympathy can be a tool to improve your relationships, and you can express yourself in the following ways:

1. EXPRESS YOUR SYMPATHY VERBALLY

Verbal expressions may be one of the most powerful ways to show sympathy but can also be tricky to execute. Try to be conscious and careful with what you say to those who are experiencing challenges in their life. Listen to what they're saying and take note of their facial expressions. In most cases, it's best to have a neutral expression on your face. That way, the person knows that you are listening without making any judgments or overreactions. When it comes to verbal expressions of sympathy, here are some essential things to keep in mind:

- **Listening is key.**

Genuine listening is one of the simple but most important things you can do for a person in a difficult situation. Sometimes, people want to talk about their circumstances and share their feelings. They may rant, vent, cry and share all the details of their troubles. It is important to avoid interrupting them or offering unsolicited advice, even if you think you know what's best for them. It's usually better to listen if you want to show sincere sympathy. The next best thing you can do is to assure the person that they can call on you if and when they need help.

- **Know the appropriate things to say.**

When it comes to expressing your sympathy through words, having a collection of phrases to say may come in handy. Just remember that every person is unique, so try and personalize your choice of words for each individual appropriately. Below are some suggestions for appropriate things you can say:

- You're always in my thoughts
- I am sorry for your loss
- I'm always here when you're ready to talk
- This must be very hard for you
- I don't know what to say, but I'm glad you could tell me
- Thank you for sharing with me. How can I help?

Make sure that you do not interrupt the person who is sharing their situation and steer clear of providing unsolicited advice. It is almost always better to listen.

- **Use a low tone when talking.**

Remember that a person who is already suffering from a difficult situation already has their emotions running high. Speaking in a low tone may help calm them down. Conversely, using a loud voice and a high-pitched tone can make them feel even more stressed. Therefore, when sharing words to express your sympathy, try speaking slowly and quietly.

2. EXPRESS YOUR SYMPATHY IN NON-VERBAL WAYS.

Perhaps you may not feel comfortable using your words to show sympathy. Or maybe, for a specific individual, you think that you need to take a different approach. For some people, showing sympathy in non-verbal ways can be extremely powerful and impactful. Try to remember that everybody is unique and responds to things differently. When it comes to non-verbal ways of showing sympathy, here are some points that are good to keep in mind:

- **Show your sympathy through physical contact.**

A simple non-verbal expression of sympathy is physical contact. A kind gesture may show support, reassurance, and concern towards the other person. Depending on how close you are with them, you can shake their hand, place your hand around their shoulders, or offer a hug. Just ensure that your physical contact is appropriate. If you notice that the person begins to feel uncomfortable or tries to move away, stop right away. Never force physical contact as the person you are supporting may take it the wrong way.

- **Consider sending a sympathy card or note.**

If you are unable to visit the person physically, sending a sympathy card or note is an excellent way to show your sympathy. For instance, if one of your friends is in another country and needs your support, it may not be ideal for you to drop everything and visit them. It is especially true if you have a job, family, and other responsibilities that you can't abandon.

If you're unable to speak with them on the phone, you can try sending them a message or letter. Even though this won't reach the person in need right away, as soon as they receive your sympathy card, they will feel your love, appreciation, and care. Verbal expressions of sympathy are usually a better option. However, if it's not possible to speak with them, a sympathy card or note can be just as impactful. Pairing a gift with your note may be suitable, depending on your relationship with them. Your gift doesn't need to be elaborate or expensive, only appropriate and relevant.

- **Let your actions convey your sympathy.**

A simple gesture or action can make all the difference to someone needing an extra hand. Always try to be specific in your offerings and make sure that you follow up with them. Practical ways of expressing sympathy could include helping around the house, meeting up with them weekly, exercising with them, or providing meals. Gestures are excellent ways to show how you are feeling. Keep in mind that no gesture is better than the other—try to be genuine and specific with what you offer.

3. CONTINUING SHOWING SYMPATHY.

When people experience a difficult situation, they often receive a wave of support from others. Unfortunately, the support that they usually receive dies down, and they may be left feeling isolated and alone. For this reason, it is critical to try and be there for them when they need it the most. Below are two things to keep in mind when showing consistent and genuine support:

- **Continue reaching out until you're sure that they are okay.**

After the person who receives support has overcome their first hurdle, try to make sure that you continue showing your support. Even after expressing your sympathy at the beginning, you can still show that you care. Keep reaching out to them, keep the connection alive, and keep offering your support. In turn, it tells them that they are not alone and that someone is there for them.

Try to do this until you are sure that the person has already overcome the issue. Even then, you can still call them once in a while to check-in. Sympathy doesn't have to end with words or gestures. You can keep on doing things to affect positive changes in their life if you care for them.

- **Make sure that you are available when the person needs you the most.**

I have already mentioned how you should assure a person who is suffering that they are in your thoughts, and they can call on you when they need help or support. This promise is a big one, and you should know what it entails. Because when the person comes knocking, you should make sure that you will be there to answer. You should be available to them when they need you. If you don't think you can commit to such a thing, it's better to find different ways to express your sympathy.

THERE ARE many ways to show sympathy to others, and mastering each will give you access to more useful tools when you need it the most. Try to keep in mind that everyone responds to acts of sympathy differently, and it is therefore essential for you to learn verbal and non-verbal ways of showing support. Either way, try and ensure that you provide proactive and consistent support and that you meet all acts of promises. Once you get it right, your genuine sympathy can have a significant impact on your life and for the lives of people around you.

PART III
WHEN SYMPATHY GOES WRONG

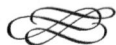

Now that you've learned more about sympathy, let me ask you a question to encourage self-reflection. Try to think about the last time someone shared an unfortunate event with you. Maybe this person experienced the death of a loved one, a loss of something important to them, or any other unfortunate circumstance. What was your immediate reaction?

Many people struggle to find the right words at that very moment. Even though sympathy is a natural response, being able to express it promptly is another story. If you have ever felt sympathetic and awkward at the same time due to a lack of words, you're not alone.

Beneficial as sympathy can be in your life; there are times when things can go south because of it. These events may negatively impact yourself and others when you don't know how to express your support in the right way.

WHAT TO AVOID WHEN SHOWING SYMPATHY TO OTHERS

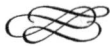

As mentioned in the previous chapter, there are many things to keep in mind when showing genuine sympathy to others. Moreover, there are a few things that you should try to avoid when expressing words or gestures of support. These are:

- **Try not to over-complicate things.**

When someone shares their perils with you, a million things may start running through your mind. You process the information they have shared, and you might start feeling bad for them. You might try to think of the best things to say or do, and so on. When you allow this to happen, things might get over-complicated. Instead, you may want to take a breath to try and clear your mind.

First, try to focus on what the other person is saying. As the feeling of sympathy washes over you, let it be. After you have listened to and understood their situation, you may start thinking about what to say. This process can make things simpler, thus, making it easier for you to express your sympathy.

• **Avoid this common statement at all costs.**

Many people think that it's okay to tell someone who has just lost a loved one that the person who has passed is "in a better place." Although we are used to this statement, and we may think that it will make the other person feel better, this isn't always the case. It is especially true if the person doesn't believe in the afterlife or different similar beliefs.

When you lose someone, you are likely to feel pain. Even if others tell you that the person you lost isn't suffering anymore, it's still painful. Often, when people try to make light of the situation, we may feel worse about it. Therefore, you may want to avoid saying this statement or others similar to it. Instead, you could say things such as, "I am sorry that you lost someone you loved so much," or something equally comforting.

• **Other common phrases to avoid.**

If you don't want to say the "wrong thing," make that that you never dismiss the things that the other person tells you. Even if you think that their emotional pain might be trivial, never express this. You may not know what they are truly going through.

Additionally, avoid saying things like "I know exactly how you're feeling," or "now you can move on," or "I don't know what I would do if someone close to me died." Statements like these are usually not received well and may put

GROW WITH SYMPATHY, EMPATHY, & COMPASSION

the other person down, and they may end up resenting you.

When you're thinking of what not to say, try to rehearse the statement in your head first. If it doesn't make you feel better, try to say it differently.

You may want to avoid these things if you are hoping to show genuine sympathy to others. If you keep these in mind, along with the other things we have already discussed, you will see that your support leads to profound recovery. Remember—the more you learn about sympathy, the more you will be able to understand it and use it appropriately. And when you can use it more appropriately, you will see better results, and you will start to grow with sympathy.

SITUATIONS WHERE YOU MAY NOT WANT TO SHOW SYMPATHY

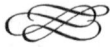

While I have spoken about sympathy in a positive light, this doesn't mean that it applies to all kinds of situations. There are also times when you should not use sympathy, and you should try to recognize such cases. Here are some of those situations where you may want to pull back and keep your thoughts, words, and gestures to yourself:

- **When you don't know the person that well ... or even at all.**

It might not be a good idea to freely express sympathy when you don't know the person very well. For instance, you are on a bus, and the person sitting next to you mentions that they were recently in a car accident. While you may say something like, "I'm sorry to hear that," or some other generic statement, it's probably not a good idea to go beyond that.

Think about what the other person would feel if you say something like, "You are always in my thoughts" or "I am here if you need me." Since you don't know each other very well, such statements might make the other person feel uncomfortable. Try to avoid these situations by expressing your sympathy appropriately when faced with people you don't know.

- **When the person expresses that they don't want your sympathy.**

Many people feel comforted when others sympathize with them. Sometimes, others may take sympathy the wrong way. They can feel like you are taking pity on them, and they may not like it. When you express sympathy to these types of people, their pain may become more severe, and the loss they have experienced may feel more intense. The more you try to talk about it, the worse the situation can become for them. And, they may take out their frustration on you and cause a rift in your relationship. These are some examples of bad things that might happen when you try to force your sympathy on those who don't want it.

In such cases, it can be better to say something simple like, "I'm here if you need me," and leave it there. If your friend wants to chat with you, at least you have provided the opportunity and awareness that you are comfortable with providing support.

Alternatively, if you know them well, you may not need to say anything to them and can go right to helping. For close friends and family, gestures may be more compelling than words. Instead of telling them that you sympathize with them, show them that you are there to help them through these difficult situations.

WHEN IT COMES to showing expressions of sympathy, try to

imagine how the other person will react. That way, you will be thinking about appropriate ways to show your support, and where your help may go wrong. Sometimes you may need to be cautious, and sometimes you may need to show tough love. Determining the right time and place to use sympathy takes practice. But once you begin mastering this skill, you will be able to adapt and show more appropriate and genuine sympathy to others.

LET YOUR WALLS DOWN, BUT LEARN TO PUT THEM BACK UP

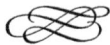

*L*earning how to protect yourself from misusers of sympathy is the final skill that I will talk about in this chapter. Unfortunately, there are many situations where people have misused sympathy. However, they may have believed it was the right thing to do. Your task is to identify these situations where others may be misusing sympathy. In turn, you will be able to protect yourself from wrongdoings as well as help others in the best way possible. Below are three situations where people misuse sympathy:

SITUATION 1: A PERSON WHO TRIES TO CONTROL YOU.

This situation can arise without you even knowing it. A person would talk to you about their problems and share just enough for you to feel bad about their situation. Then, as you express your sympathy, they build on their situation to make it seem even worse. Naturally, you may try to think of ways to make things better for them. Once you start making suggestions, this is when the person knows that they have "hooked" you.

Be very careful with people like this, as they might be experts at emotional manipulation. The more they see how willing you are to help out, the more they can find ways to control you. When you start to notice that your sympathy has led another person to start controlling your life, it's time to put a stop to your kindness. For example, if you consistently end up working overtime to finish both your task and someone else's, you may need to consider putting up your walls again. Try to explain how you are still there to support the other person and that you can help them out with simple tasks. However, you should also explain that you have your responsibilities and limitations. Try to be polite and gentle so that you don't offend the other person.

SITUATION 2: A PERSON WHO TWISTS THE FACTS TO GET SYMPATHY.

Some people are master storytellers, aside from being expert emotional manipulators. When faced with a difficult situation, and they see that they are getting sympathy, they might start twisting the facts to make their situation seem even worse. For instance, if you have a group project at school, and you discover that one of your groupmates didn't accomplish their part of the project.

When you ask them what happened, they explain that they fought with their parents the night before. This reason in itself is already good enough to explain why your group member wasn't able to do their job. However, when they see that you and your other group members are sympathizing with them, they might start twisting the facts. Your groupmate might start adding more details to their story to make things seem worse. In the end, because of how bad you and the other members of your group feel for this particular groupmate, you end up offering to do their part of the project for them.

Unfortunately, this doesn't work well for yourself and the rest of your group. You are all graded for the project, and so, you should all put an equal amount of work. Instead of doing the work for your groupmate, you may want to ask your teacher for an extension and explain the reason for it (the real reason, not any other version). That way, your groupmate can still do their work, and you would have shown sympathy but in a more appropriate way.

SITUATION 3: A PERSON WHO ALWAYS TRIES TO TAKE ADVANTAGE OF YOU.

This situation is very common for people who have something to offer, whether it be money, a special talent, a unique skill, or something equally valuable. For instance, if you are well-to-do and everybody knows it, someone might take advantage of this. For instance, if you have a friend who has a bad habit of loaning money that they aren't able to pay back, they might approach you with a sad story to make you feel bad for them.

But if your friend keeps coming back to you with the same kind of story or different versions of it, try not to let your sympathy get the best of you. Help your friend by suggesting that they avoid loaning money. Then you can teach them how to budget their money, so they don't have to keep taking loans. Give friendly suggestions on how they can increase their income. If you keep saving your friend from financial trouble because you feel bad for them, you might end up misusing sympathy. And at the same time, unconsciously enabling your friend to continue a bad habit.

As you can see through these situations, it's easy to misuse sympathy because of a lack of awareness. When you allow your feelings to take the reins, you might misuse your sympathy over and over again. Aside from your feelings, bring your mind into the equation. In turn, you will understand the situation and the person better. And it also allows you to use express sympathy properly—for your benefit and the benefit of those around you.

PART IV
WHAT IS EMPATHY?

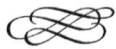

While sympathy is all about understanding the feelings that someone experiences, empathy goes a bit deeper. When you empathize with another person, you allow yourself to experience the same emotions that they are feeling. These feelings could be grief, loss, fear, or even pain. Even though you may not have experienced the same situation, you can imagine what they're going through and grasp what they are feeling.

To empathize with others, you need to try and understand what they are feeling and put yourself in their situation. Many people recognize this feeling as "putting yourself in another person's shoes." For instance, if one of your family members is feeling fearful because of a terrible accident, you may experience the same fear along with them. Or if a friend loses someone close to them, you may experience the same feelings of sadness as them. When you feel empathy, you allow yourself to tune into the emotional experiences of others. Unlike sympathy, empathy requires courage, especially since you may become vulnerable because of it. But when you can experience genuine empathy, you will start to realize how much of a gift it can be to your life—and the lives of those around you.

THE THREE MAIN TYPES OF EMPATHY

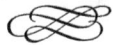

While empathy is a pretty simple concept in itself, there are many different types of empathy you can experience, which may lead to different outcomes. Knowing all of these types of empathy will equip you with the tool required to show empathy where it is most appropriate. The three main types of empathy are:

1. COGNITIVE EMPATHY

This type of empathy is also known as "perspective-taking." However, some people may not consider it as a construct of empathy. For this, you would use your mind more than your heart as you try to place yourself in the situation that someone has experienced. This way, you can see things through their perspective. Cognitive empathy—although not as warm as the other types—is a useful skill to have, especially when dealing with people in your profession.

For instance, if you're in a situation where negotiations are involved, you could put yourself in the place of the other negotiator. In doing this, you can see things through their eyes without affecting your emotions. In turn, you may be able to make smarter decisions as your feelings are less biased. Additionally, you may have a greater understanding of their perspective as well.

2. COMPASSIONATE EMPATHY

This type of empathy is the closest one to the basic definition of the term. When you experience compassionate empathy, you may feel the same emotions as another person, and these emotions would urge you to take action. Compassionate empathy is a combination of empathy and compassion. As with sympathy, compassion refers to a feeling of concern for another. However, it also involves doing something to improve the situation of the person who may need support.

Compassionate empathy can be incredibly impactful, and it is one of the best ways to express empathy. Generally, those who are seeking empathy don't want you to feel miserable with them or be too rational about their situation. Instead, they might want you to empathize with them then take action to help solve their problem. When you can do this well, you can support another person in one of the best possible ways.

3. EMOTIONAL EMPATHY

This type of empathy is the most literal as you may feel the same emotions that the other person is experiencing. You can think of it like acquiring an illness. When someone close to you is sick, and you spend time with them, you may also catch whatever they have. In the same way, you could capture the emotions of the person close to you when they share those emotions with you. Because of the nature of this type of empathy, it's also known as "emotional contagion," and it is a very emotional experience.

Among all the different types of empathy, emotional empathy is the first one we might have experienced when we were young. For instance, when a mother smiles at her baby, the baby could "catch" this emotion and smile back at her. And when a mother shows anger or disappointment, the baby may tend to feel the same way. But as adults, we might not appreciate emotional empathy as much as compassionate empathy as the latter involves taking action. After all, you might not appreciate it as much when a close friend feels miserable with you when you have a problem, compared to a friend who would try to help you out.

These are the three most common types of empathy. But there are two other types that I will share with you, as unique perspectives:

- **Somatic empathy** occurs when you feel the pain of someone else physically. For instance, if a friend is experiencing intense abdominal pain, you might end up suffering the same pain after some time. This type of empathy is quite common between twins; when one gets hurt, the other one feels the same pain too.
- **Spiritual empathy** occurs when you feel a powerful connection with a higher consciousness or a higher being. Some people consider this as enlightenment, and one of the best ways you can achieve it is through meditation.

As with sympathy, you may want to try assessing the situation first to help you determine what type of empathy to use. In some cases, the feeling of empathy would come naturally, but there may be times when you might want to take some time to think about which method to use.

HOW DOES EMPATHY DIFFER FROM SYMPATHY?

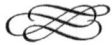

While empathy and sympathy are related to each other, they aren't the same thing. These feelings often stem from the same types of situations, but one can exist without the other. When something unfortunate happens to someone you know, you may react in three possible ways:

- You may feel bad for the person (sympathy)
- You may feel the same emotions that the person is feeling (empathy)
- You may feel bad for the person and share the same feelings they have (sympathy and empathy)

At this point, you may already have a deeper understanding of sympathy. We have previously discussed what it means, the best ways to express it, and how to avoid situations where you might end up misusing it. Given your understanding of sympathy and the definition of empathy

I have just shared, you may have a more unobstructed view of how they differ.

Another way to look at the difference between sympathy and empathy is that the former is more about understanding, whereas the latter is more about projection. You may sympathize with a person by feeling bad for them and understanding the feelings they have because of their situation. But when empathizing, you possess the ability to imagine how the other person is feeling and then feel them for yourself. Even if you don't tell the other person that you share the same feelings as them, the mere fact that you share those feelings already shows empathy.

Another term that is commonly confused with empathy is compassion-the third tool I will present to you later on. Just like empathy and sympathy, compassion is a feeling or reaction you would have when you see or hear about a person in a tough situation. If empathy is more profound than sympathy, compassion is even more profound than empathy.

Knowing how empathy differs from sympathy and compassion makes it easier to distinguish them from one another. But we're not done yet. There is still a lot to learn about empathy. And by the end of chapters 4, 5, and 6, you will understand it as deeply as sympathy (and later on, compassion).

THE SCIENCE BEHIND EMPATHY

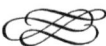

*E*mpathy occurs when you put yourself in another person's shoes, and you reach deep into your heart to experience the same emotions and feelings as them. But if you would like to experience and use genuine empathy, you may want to try to go beyond this. People who have mastered the use of empathy are known as "empaths," and they have a very high place on what's known as the "empathic spectrum." For such people, they feel the things that happen to other people in their minds and bodies. Because of this, empaths can show incredible levels of compassion to others. But being an empath can be very tiring as you may feel too much when encountering people who are facing hard times in their lives.

Although I have learned how to use empathy effectively to benefit those around me and myself in the process, I have yet to call myself an empath confidently. If you would like to develop your empathy to become an empath, you can use everything you learn here to start your journey. Be wary, though, because being an empath isn't an easy thing to do. You may have to learn how to develop strategies that safeguard yourself from all the emotions you face.

The word empathy comes from the German term "Einfühlung," meaning "feeling into." Empathy is a hot topic in the scientific world, particularly among researchers who study emotions concerning morality. One of the main reasons for this interest is that people who have little or no empathy are often combative, callous, or even "evil" in nature. Therefore, researchers want to learn how empathy truly works. This discovery could equip medical professionals with the knowledge to work with individuals that may need to become more empathetic towards themselves and others.

There are specific regions of the brain that are responsible for allowing us to feel empathy. When these regions are damaged, it may lead to a reduced level of empathy in a person. Fortunately, we can all learn to be more empathetic.

According to one study, empathy plays a vital societal and interpersonal role in our lives (Riess, 2017). Through empathy, we can share our needs, desires, and experiences. Empathy allows us to cross an emotional bridge that encourages pro-social and positive behaviors. According to the same study, having the capacity to empathize with others requires a complex interaction to occur within the neural networks in our brain. These interactions allow us to perceive the feelings and emotions of other people, connect with them both cognitively and emotionally, and imagine the perspectives of other people. And at the same time, still able to know which are our own emotions and which are the emotions of others.

Another study supports the fact that there are specific regions of the brain that play a role in how we experience empathy (Gu et al., 2012). In this study, the researchers discovered that there is more than just one region of the brain that plays a significant role in empathy. These include the anterior insula and the anterior cingulate cortex. Because of this discovery, more recent studies are focused on both the neurological and cognitive processes that affect how we feel, experience, and even use empathy.

In yet another study, the researchers suggest that there are significant neurobiological components involved when you experience empathy (Jankowiak-Siuda, Rymarczyk, & Grabowska, 2011). One thing that plays a role in this is the activation, are "mirror neurons." The presence of these neurons allows you to mimic or mirror the emotions that people have when faced with challenging situations. Neurons are only present in the empathy-related regions of the brain when no brain damage has occurred.

Another area of the brain known as the inferior frontal gyrus (IFG) plays an essential role in how we experience empathy, according to one study (Wu et al., 2018). In this study, researchers discovered that people with damaged IFG's find it challenging to recognize emotions that other people show through their facial expressions. Think about it: if you can't identify emotions, you may find it harder to express empathy.

The studies I have shared here are but a few of the many studies and researches conducted on empathy. It confirms that empathy may not be just something that happens for no reason. There are scientific explanations for empathy and knowing them may help you understand it more thoroughly. If you want to learn more about these studies and the many others out there, you might want to continue research on the topic. As you can see, it's quite fascinating – at least I think so. But for now, let's move on to the benefits that empathy can bring to yourself and others around you.

PART V
THE BENEFITS OF EMPATHY AND HOW TO BE MORE EMPATHETIC

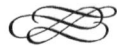

When you have empathy, it means that you can understand and share other people's emotions with them. While empathy does have science backing it up, you can look at this concept in different ways as experiencing empathy varies from one person to another. Being empathetic can be beneficial to your life in many ways. But the most significant of these benefits are:

- It allows you to establish social connections with other people. When you can imagine how other people are feeling or thinking, you may respond to their situations more appropriately.
- It helps you learn how to manage your own emotions more effectively. In doing so, you can improve your ability to deal with stressful situations without getting overwhelmed.
- It promotes positive behaviors, such as kindness. When you empathize with other people who

are in unfortunate circumstances, you may have the urge to help them out.

We all have the potential to be more empathetic, and we all experience it differently. Being able to empathize with other people can play an essential role in your social life. It can compel you to take action and make a positive change in the lives of those around you.

THE BENEFITS OF EMPATHY TO YOURSELF AND OTHERS

Having a deeper understanding of the definition of empathy allows you to experience its benefits. Empathizing with other people involves seeing a situation from their perspective and trying to imagine how they are feeling. In doing this, you will be able to share their emotions and experience these emotions alongside the person. If your empathy is strong enough, you may even go a step further by showing compassion towards people. If you're wondering how empathy can change your life, here are the benefits of empathy for you to look forward to:

- **It makes you healthier and reduces stress levels.**

Learning how to feel and use empathy is one of the best things you can do to improve your health. Surprising as this might sound, the more empathetic you are, the more you can handle stressful situations as they arise. Research shows that when you empathize with other people, you're able to create closer bonds with them. In turn, it can also help you develop healthy stress coping mechanisms. Through empathy and emotional regulation, you may notice that you don't feel as overwhelmed as you did in the past.

We all know that stress is an influential factor that may cause many diseases and illnesses. But when you don't experience stress as intensely because you're able to handle it from the get-go, you would naturally become healthier too.

- **It is an important part of survival.**

At its very core, empathy has the potential to save your life. When you can read people and situations appropriately, you might be able to make better decisions—those which will keep you safe. For instance, if a friend of yours is running with a face full of terror and tells you to run, empathy enables you to feel their fear as well.

Even without realizing it, you will be able to pick up these feelings without trying. This subconscious action can make you mentally alert and can tell you that something is wrong. Then you will be able to act appropriately to ensure that you and your friend are safe.

- **It strengthens your connections with others.**

Genuine empathy enables you to understand nonverbal cues more readily. When you are empathetic, you have the natural tendency to pay more attention to the people around you. You may even pick up the meanings of their gestures and body language. When you can do this, it becomes easier for you to recognize the thoughts of other people, thus, allowing you to respond more appropriately.

Naturally, when you can communicate more effectively with others, the connections you have with them becomes stronger. The more you can understand the feelings of other people when they experience different situations, the more you can connect with them in profound and meaningful ways. And when people see that you genuinely understand and empathize with them, they will appreciate this immensely.

- **It gives you a feeling of acceptance.**

Empathy is non-judgmental. It is a feeling and a tool that allows you to be more accepting of the thoughts, feelings, and perspectives of other people. After all, you may not be able to empathize with another person if you do not accept their feelings, thoughts, emotions, or even the people themselves. When you learn how to become more accepting of others, you will also learn how to be more accepting of yourself. And when you are more accepting of yourself, you can make positive changes in your life and for the lives of others.

- **It helps improve your professional life.**

Empathy doesn't only apply to your personal life. If you want to develop and use this skill, you may want to make it part of all aspects of your life, even in the workplace. Whether you have close relationships with your workmates or not, adding empathy to the mix might make things better. When you empathize with the people you work with, you may be able to understand them better. You may be able to see the reasons behind their actions, and you will be more willing to listen when they have something to say. Imagine if everyone in your workplace practices empathy. There would be fewer conflicts and grudges, and it may result in a more productive work environment.

- **It serves as a guide for your moral compass.**

When you experience empathy, you should try to treat other people in the same way as you expect others to treat you. Empathy allows you to establish what you consider as acceptable behaviors. Through empathy, you can create your own rules, and therefore, it can serve as a guide for your moral compass.

These six benefits are just scraping the tip of the iceberg for why you should try to be more empathic. There are so many other reasons why you should grow with empathy, and I encourage you to do your research. Write down the reasons why you would want to practice being more empathetic and notice yourself start to grow with empathy as you begin to apply it in your life. But now, let's move on to becoming a more empathetic individual.

BECOMING A MORE EMPATHETIC INDIVIDUAL

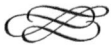

*H*aving empathy means that you can understand and feel the emotions of other people. According to neuroscientists (and some of the studies we discussed in the previous chapter), when specific regions of the brain work together, empathy occurs. The emotional side of your brain allows you to perceive other people's feelings. In contrast, the cognitive side of your brain enables you to figure out what you're feeling and how to act appropriately. While some people are more empathetic than others by nature, you can learn how to be more empathetic too. Here are some ways to do this:

- **Try putting yourself in another person's shoes.**

Cliché as this piece of advice may seem, it's quite useful. Instead of just trying another person's shoes out, try walking a mile in them too. You may also see this as trying to live another person's life to help you better understand what that person is going through. On the way, you may find out why they are feeling a certain way because of their situation.

Try this out: pick someone in your life and try to learn more about them, their habits, and their routines. Then for a few days, do the things that person does daily. This exercise can open your eyes to new experiences, and it might help you understand why that person you picked goes through their daily routine as such. In turn, this understanding can make you more open-minded and accept others more freely. The more you can accept other people and their emotions, the more empathetic you could become.

- **Learn how to really listen.**

Listening is an important skill to develop as it might help you become more sympathetic, more empathetic, and more compassionate too. But when it comes to empathy, listening to another person is one of the most effective ways to show genuine support. Try to listen with intent and focus. In turn, you may learn even more about another person's situation and how they might be feeling. While listening, you may also want to show that you understand what the other person is saying and reflect on how you are feeling. Just as sympathy, you should try and always listen first when showing genuine empathy.

- **Temporarily suspend your judgments.**

If you immediately judge another person for something that happens in their life, you may not be showing genuine empathy. Think about it: if a friend who always loses their items misplaces something valuable, how could you feel empathy if you're not surprised it happened? When a person feels judged, they might think that you don't understand them or care for them. And so when a person in distress shares their situation with you, try to suspend your judgments and just listen. It may require some practice and a conscious effort, but it's essential to developing honest empathy.

- **Use your imagination.**

Remember that empathy involves imagining what another person is going through so that you can understand and share what they are feeling. Thus, imagination is a massive part of empathy. You won't be able to experience the same event or situation as another person. So, the next best thing to do is imagine what happened, how it happened, and how it made the other person feel. Actively imagining what another person is feeling can allow you to empathize better.

- **Cultivate curiosity.**

One important characteristic of highly empathetic individuals is an insatiable curiosity, especially when it comes to strangers. Cultivating curiosity means talking to random strangers when you get a chance to or when you feel like it. For instance, you may commute to and from work each day, and you might notice a few people who share the same commuting schedule as you. Try to gather the courage to approach one of these people and strike up a conversation with them.

THINK about how easy it is for children to speak with strangers. Because they have a natural inquisitiveness, when they find something interesting about a person, they ask them about it even if that person is a stranger. Try to find this same curiosity you had when you were young so you can speak to strangers fearlessly. This curiosity that you can cultivate helps expand on your ability to show empathy as it allows you to see things from different perspectives.

EXPRESSING YOUR EMPATHY TO OTHERS

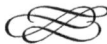

*J*ust as sympathy, there are many things to keep in mind when expressing genuine empathy to others. Now, you may want to try and show others that you care for them through expressions of empathy. As with any other skill or concept, practicing it allows you to gain mastery of it. Below are some ways to do this:

- **Focus on the needs and welfare of others.**

Empathy isn't selfish. For this tip, you may need to try using your cognitive aspect of empathy. For instance, if you see someone who is experiencing a tough situation, you may decide to empathize with this person. You may also want to try to figure out how you can help them.

Empathy doesn't just end with your feelings. After sharing the feelings of those in need, you may also want to try to think about their welfare. How can you help make their situation better? Or how can you lighten their load? Finding the answers to these questions makes you more empathetic as it allows you to go beyond your feelings and take appropriate action.

- **Try to be even more thoughtful.**

When someone is sharing their thoughts and feelings with you, try to notice your thoughts. Try to find out if you are processing what the other person is saying and not making any judgments or assumptions about it. Also, try not to think of ways to fix the other person's problems right away. As they are sharing, the most empathetic thing to do is listen. And this also shows the other person that you are thoughtful.

For instance, if a friend of yours experienced heartbreak, they may talk to you about it. The first thing you might want to do is to come to their rescue. While this seems like a noble thing to do, it might be better to listen first. Try to allow them to get their thoughts off their chest.

- **Provide physical affection when it's appropriate.**

You may not be able to show empathy through physical contact with everyone. After all, it's not the best idea to go around hugging random people when you hear about their problems. However, when it comes to the people closest to you, providing physical affection can be another great way to show empathy. Several studies have shown that physical affection can boost the levels of oxytocin in the body, thus, making you feel better.

For instance, if one of your close friends has just lost

their beloved pet, you can place your arm over their shoulders or give them a hug when they tell you the sad news. Since this person is a close friend of yours, you may already understand how much they loved their pet. Therefore, you may also be able to understand the feelings they might have because of their unfortunate situation. In this case, physical affection may be appropriate.

Always try to determine whether it's appropriate or not before making this type of gesture. In cases where you provided physical affection, and it makes the other person feel uncomfortable, stop, and apologize. Then try to think of different ways to express your empathy.

- **Offer help.**

When you empathize with someone, the next thing you can do is offer to help them out. It shows the other person that you have listened to them, understood their situation, and that you want to make them feel better by doing something to help. For instance, if you're in school and you see one of your friends struggling with one of your subjects, you can offer to help your friend out with things. It doesn't even have to be with schoolwork. As long as the things you do take some pressure off your friend, they will appreciate it.

Offering help is a beautiful act of empathy. It shows your willingness to give the other person your time to make life easier for them. And you may want to do this even without asking for anything in return. The mere act of offering can also be considered a gesture of empathy. Whether the person takes you up on your offer or not, at least you reached out to help.

- **Talk to other people, even if you don't know them very well.**

Many people may know that curiosity is an essential aspect of empathy. Think about it: how could you imagine what a person feels if you don't ask them what happened? It's quite challenging to genuinely empathize with others when you may not be aware of their entire situation. But if you try to talk to other people, you may understand why they feel this way.

To develop your empathy further, you might want to try talking to people you don't know, too. Start with small talk then try asking more profound questions. For instance, you could ask them what their day-to-day lives are like, how they are doing right now, and more. Your deeper connection allows you to see things from different perspectives. And when something unfortunate happens to someone that you know, you may be able to understand them and empathize faster after exposing yourself to different kinds of people through communication.

- **Practice empathy whenever you can.**

To become a master of empathy, you can practice and cultivate this ability. All of the tips I have shared may help you become a more empathetic person. Try applying these strategies to your life so that you can practice as much as you can. With enough practice, you might be on your way to being an empath. Even if this isn't your goal, practicing still makes you a better person because it makes empathy one of your go-to tools when supporting other people.

EMPATHY, although we all have the potential for it, is still an uncommon trait. But cultivating it is important, especially if you would like to use it as a tool for positive change in your life and the lives of those closest to you. When you express empathy, this can help you create genuine connections with other people. And when people see you as an empathetic person, they know that coming to you will make them feel understood, valued, and respected.

PART VI
WHEN EMPATHY WORKS AGAINST YOU

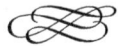

Empathy is an important skill and tool that can play a significant role in bringing people closer together. Empathy can be the sadness you feel when a friend loses a loved one. And, it can also be the happiness you feel when a friend walks down the aisle to marry their partner.

However, empathy isn't always positive.

Just like sympathy (and compassion later on), empathy has a downside. In particular, when you empathize too much, you might get consumed by the feelings you share with another person. And when this happens, you might end up neglecting your own emotions or needs. When you empathize too much—especially the negative emotions—you may become more susceptible to anxiety, depression, and other byproducts.

Empathy can be a beautiful thing as it can offer several benefits to your life. But it's essential to how to use it properly to help you learn how to protect yourself from being too empathetic towards others.

WHAT HAPPENS WHEN YOU MISUSE EMPATHY?

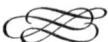

Knowing when to use empathy or when to avoid it is something that you will learn through practice. Most times, it is appropriate to sense what others are feeling. However, when you experience negative feelings for long periods, these emotions might start manifesting in your body. When this happens, you may begin to feel other people's pain, both physically and emotionally, at an uncontrolled rate. These are the things that could happen to you if you misuse empathy:

- **Empathetic reactivity leads to stress and burnout.**

Empathetic reactivity can cause your body to produce high levels of cortisol, the stress hormone. In turn, you may find it more difficult to release negative emotions. Normal levels of empathy can make positive changes in your life and for the people around you. However, taking on the feelings and experiences of others too intensely might leave you feeling hopeless, anxious, or depressed.

Over time, this might cause you to get burned out, especially if you aren't able to help other people overcome their problems. Once you start feeling burned out, you may want to stop empathizing for a while. Try to take some time for yourself, and think of other creative ways to help, as empathy isn't always the answer.

- **Empathy shapes and misguides your feelings.**

Experiencing empathy-based guilt frequently may have a detrimental effect on your wellbeing. For instance, you may see homeless people on the streets and empathize with them. Although you may not be responsible for the situations they are in, you may feel some level of guilt. Because of this, you might start giving away your money and possessions to them to make them feel better.

YOUR KINDNESS MAY BECOME a habit that makes you feel better for those in need. But if you share your acts of kindness too much, you may find yourself in a tricky situation. It's okay to empathize with strangers. But it's not advisable to allow empathy to sweep you away from reality so much that it leaves you in a tight situation. After all, you may not be able to help others if you are the one needing help. If you feel like you're losing yourself, try to take a step back and focus on yourself for a while. When you start to feel better, you could then try empathizing with other people again.

IMPORTANT THINGS TO KEEP IN MIND WITH SHOWING EMPATHY TO OTHERS

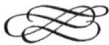

Useful as empathy can be to your life, it's also helpful to know when you don't have to be empathetic towards other people. This understanding is an important aspect of empathy as it allows you to use this tool in the best and most appropriate ways possible. To help you out, here are a few more pointers to help you ensure that your empathy is genuine:

- **Empathizing doesn't mean forcing your own emotions on others.**

Empathizing with others means that you are the one sharing the other person's emotions. It doesn't always work the other way around. For instance, a coworker may tell you about a mistake that they made at work and how they felt about it. Try to avoid making the conversation about yourself and avoid sharing a similar experience that you may have encountered previously. Try to remember that we are all unique and different from one another. Even if the same mistake didn't make you feel bad in the past, your coworker might feel devastated when it happened to them. Genuine empathy means focusing on others, not forcing other people to focus on you.

- **Learn how to cultivate non-reactive empathy.**

Reactive empathy is one of the most intense kinds of empathy to experience as it tends to make you lose yourself in the process. For this reason, you may want to learn how to cultivate non-reactive empathy. To do this well, try to make yourself more aware of the thoughts and feelings that arise within you. The more aware you are of these feelings, the more non-reactive you can be. Try to name these thoughts and emotions and learn to accept them. Then remember that these aren't your own. These are the thoughts and emotions you share with the other person.

Instead of fighting or resisting these emotions, accepting them and identifying them could make you feel less overwhelmed. This awareness may also allow you to make a clearer distinction between your thoughts and emotions and those of other people. If you're looking for non-destructive ways to empathize with others, this might be an approach that's worth considering.

- **Try not to empathize with too many people at once.**

Many people find it hard to empathize with more than one person at a time. Since empathy involves sharing the same emotions of another, it's not easy to do this when there are two people in front of you. It is particularly tricky as they may have different experiences and emotions from one another.

GROW WITH SYMPATHY, EMPATHY, & COMPASSION

. . .

As HUMAN BEINGS, our minds and hearts may not be able to hold a wide range of emotions at the same time. Instead, you might want to learn how to manage your empathy, so you don't end up running around trying to empathize with too many people at once. When you start to focus on one problem at a time, your empathy will be more direct, impactful, and appropriate for the given situation.

The bottom line is that empathy, while beneficial, doesn't belong everywhere. As you learn how to use empathy more effectively, you might also want to learn how to gauge the situations and people you encounter. In turn, you will improve your ability to determine when empathy isn't appropriate.

SITUATIONS WHERE YOU SHOULD AVOID USING EMPATHY

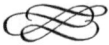

Useful as empathy can be, it's also helpful to know when you may not need to be empathetic towards other people. Understanding these situations may help you avoid using empathy where it isn't required. Here are a few pointers with examples:

- **Sometimes, people are too deep in their problems.**

Empathy may not be appropriate in situations that are already dire and hopeless. For instance, if one of your friends is feeling down and they come to you with a problem, empathizing with them might lead to destructive results. In turn, you may feel their pain and not be in a position to offer support. For this situation, it might be more appropriate to use sympathy or compassion instead. That way, you can be there to listen and help where you can.

- **Not all people want to be the object of another person's empathy.**

When you see someone in deep thought with a sad or pained look on their face, try not to approach them right away. And even if you do want to help this person, try not to come on too strong. Just because a person may look miserable, it doesn't mean that they are inviting you to empathize with them. Instead of empathizing right away, you may want to gently ask the person if everything is okay or see if they ready to talk. Try to give them space and allow them to share their thoughts. Depending on how they respond, you can decide on what the most appropriate way is to offer help.

- **When it makes other people feel bad, stop.**

When people see that their pain might be causing others to feel pain, this might make them feel even worse. For instance, if one of your parents is sick and in constant pain, they might feel worse if they see you suffering too. Instead, you may want to show that you support them and that you can be strong for them. In cases where your empathy is hurting those you love, it might be better to show strength and love.

- **If you're unsure what to feel, then listen.**

The basic concept of empathy is to be able to share another person's feelings. But what if you have never experienced the same thing that they have? How can you genuinely empathize with them? For instance, a close friend of yours might have broken up with their partner, and you may have never been in a romantic relationship before. It might not be easy for you to try and imagine what they are feeling.

In cases like these, you may express your empathy by listening and being there for the other person. Rather than trying to share their emotions but coming up short or insincere, listening might be the better option.

WHEN YOU LEARN how and when to use empathy, this makes it even more powerful. And when you master empathy, it can be one of your superpowers! Just like sympathy, empathy is a valuable tool to change the lives of people and even yourself! But we are not done yet. I have one last means to share with you, and this might be the most powerful one of all.

PART VII
WHAT IS COMPASSION?

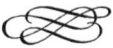

Compassion is pure, beautiful, and it applies to all people, whether you know them or not. While sympathy and empathy are all about understanding and sharing the emotions of other people, compassion is all about translating those emotions–and your love for the person–into action. Simply put, compassion means 'to suffer together,' so much that you will feel a sense of motivation to relieve any negative feelings that someone may have. It refers to your capacity and willingness to stand alongside another person and prioritize their needs before your own.

If one of your goals is to live a more compassionate life, you may have to change a few of your habits with practice, persistence, and self-motivation. Don't worry, though, because you can improve your understanding by learning more about the fundamentals of compassion and how to apply them—some of which I will share with you later on. As with the other two tools we have already discussed, compassion comes with its benefits. But, first, we must understand what compassion truly means.

DEFINING COMPASSION

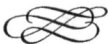

When you look at the literal definition of compassion, it means "to suffer together." This feeling is a profound experience as it brings much positivity even though it starts from a negative experience. According to emotion researchers, compassion is a feeling that emerges when you encounter another person who is suffering. Then you would feel the urge to help ease that suffering any way you can.

With these definitions, it's clear that compassion is neither sympathy or empathy. Nevertheless, these feelings and essential tools for life are all related. Compassion goes beyond sympathy and empathy, as you may feel a desire to help those in need. It's also important to note that compassion differs from altruism. The latter refers to selfless and kind behaviors that you would do because you feel compassion for another person. However, you may still feel compassion towards someone else but not act on it. And compassion isn't the only thing that would motivate you to do something altruistic.

Compassion is a wonderful thing, but many, mostly cynics, dismiss this emotion as irrational, "touchy-feely," or even useless. But those who do believe in compassion (like me) see it as something more. To deepen our understanding of compassion, researchers have tried to map out its biological basis, thus, allowing them to provide a suggestion of its evolutionary purpose. According to different research and studies, when you experience compassion, your heart rate starts slowing down. Then your body secretes oxytocin, which is also known as the "bonding hormone." After that, the regions of the brain responsible for pleasurable feelings, caregiving, and even empathy, are activated. This activation, in turn, urges you to approach those who are suffering and offer your help or support.

Compassion is a powerful motivating force that can move you to help other people mentally, emotionally, and physically. Even if helping them isn't easy, you might still feel motivated to do it. When you feel compassion, you may also have a sensitivity to those who are in need, suffering, or facing challenges. In Latin, the etymology of the term compassion means "co-suffering." This definition brings it closer to empathy, as you would feel for others. But compassion runs deeper as you would do something to ease the negative feelings of another person.

When you feel compassion towards another person, you would feel moved by the situation they are in and the feelings they are experiencing. Because of this, you may want to either help out or even solve their problems for them. Acts of compassion are often characterized by helpfulness, while the qualities of compassion are kindness, patience, perseverance, and warmth. It's very challenging to be compassionate while being judgmental or angry at the person. Compassionate acts focus more on caring as you try to improve another person's situation. And for this reason, compassion is considered as one of the greatest virtues you can have in life.

HOW COMPASSION DIFFERS FROM SYMPATHY AND EMPATHY

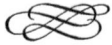

Compassion is more profound than sympathy and empathy as you would go beyond your feelings and act upon them. When you feel compassion, you would understand their pain (sympathy), feel their pain (empathize with them), and try to help them out of their difficult situation. Compassion means facing challenges instead of running away from them. It can be extremely challenging to see those you love in pain. However, with compassion, you may not allow yourself to get overwhelmed, nor would you ignore the fact that they are suffering. Practicing compassion means being there for those you love. Putting in the time and effort to make a difference in their lives. Compared to sympathy and empathy, compassion is a more complex process as it involves a few steps:

- First, you become aware of another person's situation.
- Then you would feel sympathetic concern for the person because you are emotionally affected

GROW WITH SYMPATHY, EMPATHY, & COMPASSION

by their situation. Sometimes, you would even go as far as sharing the pain the other person is feeling.
- Next, you would feel an urge to help so that the other person won't suffer anymore.
- Finally, you would respond to their situation by offering your help or support to ease the other person's suffering.

While compassion may seem like a complex thing, it can also be very simple and pure. For instance, the mere act of listening to another person can qualify as an act of compassion, especially if being heard already makes the other person feel better.

We have already discussed the meaning of sympathy. When you sympathize with another person, you understand and accept the feelings they have because of their situation. Sometimes, you might feel the urge to take action, but it won't go as far as trying to help them overcome their challenges. Instead, you might try to comfort them and make them feel better through your words and gestures.

We have already discussed the meaning of empathy, as well. When you empathize with another person, you share their feelings. As you have learned, empathy can be dangerous, especially if you don't know when to use it, and when it's time to detach yourself from another person's emotions. When this happens, you might end up feeling burned out as you cannot continue sharing negative emotions with other people. Unlike empathy, compassion is renewable when you can empathize with others but also help them feel better; the likelihood of getting burned out decreases.

When you perform compassionate acts, you experience

something more profound. You would feel a stronger connection with the person you help even though you may not get anything in return from the help you provide. Being compassionate doesn't mean that you see other people as weak or as victims. Instead, you would see them as human just like you, and you take steps to empower and support them to ease their troubles.

Let me share with you a situation that may help you understand compassion better. Try to imagine two friends —Mary and Linda—where Mary fell into a well, and Linda wants to help her because she feels compassion. From the position Linda is in, she has a good perspective of how Mary can get herself out of the well. Although Linda may feel the panic Mary is feeling, she doesn't succumb to it. Instead, she remains present and rational for Mary so that she can offer suggestions to get out of the well. Once Linda can help Mary out of the well, they both come out feeling better because Mary is now out of her dire situation.

Now, let's try to see how different the situation will turn out when Linda uses sympathy or empathy instead of compassion:

- **When Linda feels sympathy for Mary.**

In the same situation, Linda would be able to understand how Mary is feeling. After all, who wants to get stuck in a well? Linda would feel bad for Mary and try to make her feel better by offering comforting words. Unfortunately, in such a situation, words aren't enough. While panicking and feeling foolish for falling into the well in the first place, Mary might end up feeling like a victim to a bad situation. In turn, this victimization might make her feel even worse.

GROW WITH SYMPATHY, EMPATHY, & COMPASSION

- **When Linda feels empathy for Mary.**

Given the same situation once again, Linda will not only understand Mary's situation, but she will share her feelings too. While this might make Mary feel better for a while since she knows that someone is acknowledging and sharing her feelings, she would still be stuck in the well. Much as Linda empathizes with Mary, the lack of action doesn't solve the problem.

Now, this is where compassion comes in. Aside from understanding and feeling the emotions of another, you could make a conscious decision to help. Through compassion, you have the drive to take action to help the person in need. Although this example isn't a very common situation, it clearly illustrates how these three tools work. It also shows how, in some situations, it's not enough to sympathize or empathize with another person. When the situation calls for it, you may also show compassion towards others to help them through difficult situations.

Let me share another example with you; it's one most of us have experienced at least once in our lives. For this example, two friends—Winter and Carmen—talk about how one of Carmen's siblings has recently passed away. In such a situation, sympathy, empathy, and compassion are all appropriate, but they will lead to different outcomes:

- **When Winter feels sympathy for Carmen**

Given this situation, Winter may provide Carmen with comforting words. Winter would feel bad about Carmen's situation and would try to show her support through words or gestures that she deems appropriate for the situation.

- **When Winter feels empathy for Carmen**

Given this situation, Winter will feel the same pain Carmen is feeling and may shed tears along with her friend. Such a case would happen if Winter and Carmen were close, and Winter knew Carmen's sister too. Through empathy, Winter will be able to imagine the pain Carmen is feeling, and she would share that pain with her.

- **When Winter feels compassion for Carmen**

Given the same situation, Winter will sympathize with Carmen, empathize with her, and try to do something to ease the pain her friend is feeling. For instance, she can volunteer to take care of an important task like the catering services for the funeral. After comforting Carmen, Winter will try to find ways to make her friend feel better. Concrete, practical ways that will make a difference. In turn, this is what compassion is all about.

ONE OF THE best things about compassion is that it allows you to care for other people without losing yourself in the process. This may happen because it is possible to feel compassionate without empathizing with another person. More often than not, though, you may have to feel some level of sympathy for another person for it to lead to compassion.

THE SCIENCE BEHIND COMPASSION

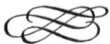

Many people confuse compassion with empathy. According to researchers, empathy is emotionally or viscerally experiencing the feelings of another person. Empathy is also like "mirroring" another person's emotions as you would feel the same way as them. While compassion may involve an empathetic response, it also involves a genuine desire to help the other person.

Compassion is not an imaginary experience or emotion. More and more evidence from research and studies have suggested that, at our very core, we as human beings have a "compassionate instinct." For this reason, compassion is innate as it already exists within us. Some researchers even say that responding to situations with compassion is both automatic and natural, and it can contribute to your survival.

One particularly interesting study showed that rats could show compassion to one another (Mason et al., 2011). In the study, rats showed compassion by going out of their way to save other rats, even though they had an opportunity to gorge on chocolate. Other similar studies done on other animals have shown similar results as well. For instance, another study focused on chimpanzees and young children (Warneken et al., 2007). In this study, the researchers discovered how these two mammals (despite being of different species) tend to help each other out even if they have to overcome obstacles first.

Another interesting study worth taking note of at Harvard (Rand et al., 2012) focused on human beings, both children and adults. In this study, the researchers concluded that the very first impulse of people of all ages is to show compassion by helping others. However, the difference is that some adults might feel worried about how other people will interpret this impulse. Because of this, their feeling of worry may hinder their impulse to help out. Still, it's good to know that compassion is a strong and natural impulse we all have.

When you think about it, learning that compassion is an innate tendency isn't that surprising. After all, compassion is essential for our survival. Think about it: when an entire community of people shows compassion towards each other, won't they survive and thrive better than a community of people who try to take advantage of each other every chance they get? The more compassionate we are towards others, the more we can help each other survive. Even in dangerous situations, being able to show compassion means that more of us will make it out alive compared to when we all have an "every man for himself" mentality.

Compassion is truly a real thing as it also occurs in our brains, as explained by another study (Rajmohan & Mohandas, 2007). According to this study, there is a specialized group of cells in our brains that stimulate compassion. We all have these cells, and they allow us to mirror the emotions of other people. And when you can do this, you will feel the urge to help, especially when the emotions that you mirror cause you to feel distressed. Aside from feeling good after doing something to help ease another person's pain (as well as your own), compassion also offers other health benefits.

The more compassionate you are, the more beneficial it is to your overall mental and physical health. Showing compassion makes you feel more positive about life. And when you can connect with others in positive and meaningful ways, this can even help give your physical health a boost (Park et al., 2014). This, in turn, helps you recover faster from illnesses and diseases. There is even research that shows how compassion and positivity can potentially extend your lifespan (Brown et al., 2011).

One of the most important reasons why living a more compassionate life is that the mere act of helping or giving to others can feel just as good as being the recipient of these compassionate acts. Sometimes, it can even make you feel even better, especially when you can help those you love the most. When you feel happy by making others happy, this activates the "pleasure centers" of your brain, thus, making you feel healthier too. Think about it: do you feel better when you buy something for yourself or when you give something to someone in need, and you see that this makes them happier? If you're a compassionate person, the latter will move you more than the former. So, when you start feeling this way, you would know that you are already becoming more compassionate as a person.

PART VIII
THE BENEFITS OF COMPASSION AND HOW TO LEAD A MORE COMPASSIONATE LIFE

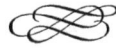

Since compassion means "to suffer with others," it can feel like empathy since you would somehow feel another person's sadness, suffering, or pain. As soon as you take action to help another, you have already gone beyond sympathy and empathy as you would have already transitioned into compassion. Action is the main component that sets compassion apart from other feelings like concern, sensitivity, commiseration, and even pity. When you're compassionate about someone, you get involved in their life. Sometimes, you would even act on behalf of the person who is suffering.

According to research, there is a neurological basis for feeling compassion towards another person. As with empathy, there are specific regions in our brains that get activated when you feel compassion. Because of this neurological aspect of compassion, you may experience several good things:

- When you feel compassion, your heart rate tends to slow down, counteracting any physical manifestations of stress that you might be experiencing.
- Compassion can also reduce the stress you feel. Although you would start by feeling bad or stressed about another person's situation, when you do something to make that situation better, you are also alleviating the stress that comes with the situation. And this beneficial effect happens to you and the person you helped.
- As we've discussed, showing compassion towards other people will make you feel good. Taking action and seeing the good you have done activates the pleasure centers of your brain. This also has a wonderful effect on your self-esteem.
- The more compassionate you are, the more you will be able to inspire others to be compassionate too. And when more people show compassion instead of anger, detachment, or cynicism, they will feel the urge to help others out too. When this happens, you will see an improvement in your community as a whole. Because of compassion, you will all be able to live happier lives. (We'll talk a little more about how this works in the next section.)

Being the final tool we're discussing in this book, I truly think compassion is the most profound. After mastering sympathy and empathy, you would have already prepared yourself to live a more compassionate life. With these three tools, you will be able to genuinely care for others in ways you have never even though of before. Over time, you will start experiencing the wonderful benefits of compassion in your life too...

WHAT ARE THE BENEFITS OF BEING COMPASSIONATE?

Compassion is as important to our lives as the food we eat, the clothes on our backs, and the air that we breathe. Without compassion, our world might spiral into something completely different. Without compassion, we would not be able to look up to great people such as Nelson Mandela, Mother Teresa, Mahatma Gandhi, Martin Luther King, Jr., and others. And without compassion, you might not be able to create deep connections with the people in your life. Compassion is a highly beneficial experience, feeling, characteristic, and tool. By being more compassionate, you may look forward to the following benefits to your world and community:

- **Compassion may increase your happiness and overall well-being.**

By helping others, you will learn more about yourself, grow with compassion, and also feel good because of your positive impact on another person.

- **Compassion can also help other people's happiness and overall well-being.**

When you combine compassion and optimism, this could be beneficial for all people, especially those who are prone to anxiety, depression, and other negative emotions. You may pull people out of a rut and, through genuine compassion, have a profound and positive impact on people's lives.

- **Compassion opens your mind and your heart.**

It broadens your perspective while helping you discover your true identity. Compassion shows your commonality with other people so that you can realize that they are suffering as well, just like you. Because of this, you will feel motivated to help others and yourself in the process.

- **Compassion strengthens social connections between people.**

Social connections are essential in our lives as these improve our ability to relate, our self-worth, and even our communication skills. When you live a compassionate life, you are also allowing yourself to become more profoundly connected with other people. This energy inspires commitment and loyalty, thus, giving you a strong support system that you can rely on in times of need.

- **Compassion improves relationships within families.**

Compassion encourages positive parenting so that children can grow in a home with love, positivity, and genuine care. In turn, the children learn these vital skills to flourish and grow with compassion.

- **Compassion can potentially improve your health by making your immune system stronger.**

Some studies have found that compassion also helps you recover from illnesses more rapidly, and it can even extend your lifespan.

- **Compassion can improve commitment in school.**

In the educational setting, when teachers show compassion to each other and the other members of the school, there is an increase in organizational commitment, job satisfaction, and overall motivation. When teachers show compassion to their students, this leads to better learning and an increase in cooperation and interaction from the students.

- **Compassion leads to the regrounding of oneself.**

Practicing self-compassion allows you to understand yourself more profoundly as you find ways to help others who are in need. Unlike empathy, compassion can help reduce the risk of burnout as you would be relieving your stress by helping those you love out of difficult situations. Self-compassion can also help combat the negative effects of stress. One of the most significant effects of this benefit is that it leads to positive aging. If you have ever heard the phrase "aging gracefully," this may especially apply to people who live compassionate lives.

- **Compassion helps to mitigate situations.**

When you encounter conflicts in your life, compassion can help facilitate peace and reconciliation. Showing compassion to the person you conflict with shows them that you still care about them despite your current situation. This support, in turn, may inspire them to show the same kind of compassion towards you and others around them.

If there is anything in the world that should be contagious, it's compassion. With all the benefits compassion offers, spreading it to those around you and the rest of the world may promote a richer, more fulfilling life for all of us. Now, it's time to find out when you should be using compassion.

WHEN SHOULD COMPASSION BE USED?

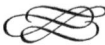

Compassion is a wonderful emotion that is deeply rooted in our minds, and it involves both motivation and intentionality. Most situations that involve people in need or those suffering from difficulties require compassion. And if you want to live a more compassionate life, you may want to practice it as frequently as you can. To do this, you need a change of mindset to help you understand that showing compassion is a choice. The emotions you might feel towards another person when you find out that they are suffering might come naturally. However, it is your choice to take action to make that person's situation better.

Therefore, to live a life of compassion, you may have to work to make it part of your life consciously. As with any new concept or skill, the more you use compassion, the more it comes naturally to you. If you want to be more compassionate, you may want to choose one of your fundamental motivational systems for caring. Then you can cultivate this to help it grow and come more naturally. In doing this, your brain changes, thus, allowing you to take more control of your feelings, thoughts, and actions.

As I have mentioned in the beginning, you can use compassion in virtually any kind of situation. As long as it doesn't push you to do something dangerous, illegal or hurtful, you can show compassion to those around you— even if it's not the easiest thing in the world to do. For instance, if someone you dislike immensely has fallen into a dire situation, you can either choose to ignore them or show compassion. But when you see them struggling, sympathy or empathy might come knocking. You might feel bad for the person, even if you don't like them. Then comes the choice of whether or not you will help out. I believe that if you want to live a more compassionate life, it's better to help.

In moments where you see other people in need, this would be the best time to set aside your judgments and negativities. Remember that we are all human beings who, at one point in our lives, will find ourselves struggling with life. And when you are the one who bears witness to such events, you could also be the one to extend a compassionate hand to help. Cultivating compassion makes it easier for you to use it as needed.

Your capacity for healing increases, and so does your motivation to help others. Of course, this doesn't mean that you aren't allowed to turn down people in need because there will always be situations when you would have to say no. For instance, you should try not to put yourself in danger to help others out, nor should you put other people in danger to solve another person's problem. As with sympathy and empathy, you need to determine what kind of reaction the situation calls for. Identifying these situations may be a challenge in the beginning, but keep practicing, and you're sure to learn how to use compassion as a tool for positive change.

HOW TO LEAD A MORE COMPASSIONATE LIFE

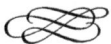

Compassion is something you can practice to bring long-term happiness and fulfillment into your life. This isn't about immediate gratification (although you will feel great when you see the good effects of your good deeds). Instead, it's more about being able to find true, lasting happiness by making positive changes in your life and the lives of those around you. There are many things you can do to lead a more compassionate life. Here are some of the simplest yet most effective ways I have learned from all my experience:

- **Create a morning ritual that inspires you to be more compassionate.**

When you start your day with compassion, this sets the tone for everything else you do. Therefore, one thing you can do to start becoming more compassionate is to create your morning ritual from the moment you open your eyes. I start each day with a simple mantra. When I wake up, I stretch, breathe deeply, and express my gratitude for a new day. Then I say something along the lines of "Today, I am grateful for being alive, and I will express this gratitude by being more compassionate to others." You can come up with your mantra that you can either say out loud or in your mind. Simple as this practice is, it will do wonders for your inspiration.

- **Try to be more humble and selfless.**

A compassionate life doesn't include pride or boasting. When you do something compassionate for another person, you don't have to brag about it. And it's not appropriate to show compassion to others to impress either. Compassion is more about being humble and selfless. When you feel bad for someone, and you genuinely want to improve their situation, you could do something about it. While you do, try not to think about what you will get out of your actions, but what good you will bring to the lives of those you show compassion to.

- **Search for commonalities.**

For many people, they aren't able to show compassion because they see themselves as different from others. For instance, if you aren't that rich and you see someone—whom you know is rich—struggling with a problem. However, you might feel bad for the person; you focus on how different you are in terms of status that you end up ignoring them. But if you want to practice compassion, try to search for the things you have in common with others instead of focusing on what makes you different. For instance, you can say things to yourself like:

GROW WITH SYMPATHY, EMPATHY, & COMPASSION

1. This person wants to find happiness, just like me.
2. This person is suffering just as I had suffered in the past.
3. This person needs support because their situation is just like what I've experienced.

Focusing on your commonalities makes it easier for you to feel compassion towards others and take action because of what you are feeling. It also makes compassion emerge more naturally when you are faced with people who are struggling in their lives.

- **Empathize with others and let this motivate you to do something about it.**

When a person is feeling pain, try to feel their pain as well. When a person is feeling sorrow because they lost someone, they love, try to feel their sorrow too. Use your empathy to motivate you, to encourage you to do something to make the other person's situation lighter, easier, or more bearable. And when they feel joy because of what you did for them, try to feel that joy as well. Empathy can be a powerful motivator for compassion when you learn how to use it properly.

- **Instead of judging, try to learn how to accept and forgive.**

When you judge others who are suffering, compassion will go out the window. How can you feel compassion for someone when judgments cloud your thoughts? Instead of judging, try to learn how to accept others more. Accept the person, accept the situation they are in, and accept the feelings they have towards their current situation. Even if the person has wronged you, try to accept them by learning how to forgive as well.

There will be times when you may encounter people who make you so angry or frustrated because you know that they are in a difficult situation because of their actions. If you want to show such people compassion, forgive them first. Forgive them for what they did or said to you and forgive them for doing things that have now placed them in harm, pain, or suffering. Only when you can forgive and accept will you be able to open your heart to compassion.

- **Be kind always.**

Again, another simple tip for you. But you might be surprised at how difficult this can be. If you weren't particularly compassionate in the past, being kind to others may seem strange at first. Instead of gossiping about other people's problems or feeling bad for them, you will be too busy being kind. This means that you open your heart to those who are suffering and show them genuine compassion. Sometimes, you don't even need a huge gesture. Something as simple as listening and offering heartfelt words can immediately make people feel better. So, if you want to lead a more compassionate life, be kind!

As you may have noticed, these tips are simple, easy to understand, and doable. But they're not mastered overnight, so instead, be patient with yourself. I've struggled with one or two of these tips, but stuck with them and continue to develop these skills.

GROW WITH SYMPATHY, EMPATHY, & COMPASSION

But we're not done yet; there are other things you can do to incorporate compassion into your daily life. This will make it easier for you to use it whenever the situation calls for it.

COMPASSION IN DAILY LIFE

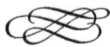

To make compassion part of your life, try practicing it daily. Doing this builds momentum until you have incorporated this positive habit into your life. Furthermore, compassion in daily life also allows you to experience life fully instead of just standing on the sidelines. Trust me; compassion will change your life. And when you use it as a tool for change, the wonderful effects will snowball even more... in a good way! Here are some things you can do to incorporate compassion into your daily life:

- **Try to say "thank you" more often.**

In the previous section, the first tip I shared with you involved expressing gratitude at the start of each day. Aside from this, you may want to practice saying "thank you" whenever something good happens to you or whenever someone does something good for you. Feeling grateful for life makes it easier to show compassion to others. When you consciously recognize the things in your life to feel grateful for, you will feel more inspired to reach out to others, especially when you think they need help.

- **Learn how to appreciate and trust others more.**

For this, you can start with the people closest to you. Sadly, we often fall into the trap of taking people for granted. And when something bad happens to them, we always assume that they will be able to pick themselves up, especially if we know that they are strong people. But what if they can't? What if they have been waiting for someone to show them some compassion, so they find a reason to overcome their problems? What if you had the chance to help, but you didn't?

You might not have to worry about these things if you learn how to appreciate and trust others more. Think about it: when you consciously make an effort to appreciate a friend and show that appreciation, wouldn't it be easier to show them compassion when something bad comes their way? Yes, it will be. Appreciation and trust are related to compassion, and both of these could help you become more compassionate in your daily life.

- **Motivate other people and give them hope.**

As I have mentioned, compassion doesn't always have to come with a huge gesture. It could be as simple as giving encouraging words to another person to motivate them and give them hope. Whenever you encounter others, try saying kind words to them. You don't know whose day you will brighten up by doing this. And the best part is that it costs you absolutely nothing! Make it a habit to say kind things to other people, especially when you think they need a bit of motivation. And when people start saying nice things back, you will also feel your hope rising within you.

- **Genuinely show your support to other people.**

Often, people can find themselves in hopeless situations because they feel like they are isolated, and they have nobody to turn to. For such people, the most meaningful act of compassion can come in the form of support. It could be about an impossible dream, a difficult problem, a devastating heartbreak, or a serious illness. By showing your genuine support to another person, it will make you a more compassionate person.

- **Give other people your time and attention.**

Another excellent way to incorporate compassion into your daily life is by spending quality time with others. I don't mean just being in the same room with a person in need but focusing on other things. Give other people your time and undivided attention. This makes them feel valued, and it shows them how important they are to you. This is one of the greatest acts of compassion you could do, especially in this modern-day world where we seem to be living too far apart from each other.

- **Show compassion to yourself, too.**

Self-compassion is essential if you want this virtue to be part of your life. When you are the one faced with issues, try applying all of these steps you have learned thus far (and everything else you will learn) toward yourself. That way, you won't have to spiral down into darkness and hopelessness. Instead, you may learn how to give yourself hope and motivate yourself to keep moving forward through compassion. Besides, the more compassionate you are to yourself, the easier it becomes to show compassion to others.

COMPASSION DOESN'T HAVE to be a difficult thing. It may seem unfamiliar and challenging at first, but once you see the wonderful effects it may have on your life, you might realize that it is all worth it. So, try a little compassion and see how big of a difference it will make in your life!

PART IX
THE DOWNSIDE OF COMPASSION

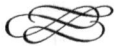

Although compassion is a noble thing, there may come a time when your decision to act compassionately hurts someone else. Whether you are showing compassion to yourself or someone in need, taking action to help make the situation better might cause problems for another. So, what do you do in such a situation? Do you stick with your decision to act compassionately and risk the feelings of someone else? Or do you give up your compassionate quest, so you don't end up hurting another person in the process?

Just like sympathy and empathy, compassion isn't perfect as it has its downsides. For instance, if one of your coworkers is swamped with work and has a breakdown because they can't handle all the tasks for the day, you might feel compassion for them. This feeling might give you an urge to take action even if you know that you also have many tasks to finish. But if your coworker's tasks are already overdue while you still have time to finish your work, you might choose to help them out. But then, because you helped your coworker, you end up too tired to finish your tasks. Then you realize that now you are the one experiencing a delay.

In this situation, the person who ended up compromised because of your compassionate action was yourself. Because of this, you might end up feeling frustrated or guilty, even though you started with good intentions. And when you see that your coworker is doing fine while you are the one struggling, you might even end up feeling resentful. Fortunately, compassion begets compassion. Thus, your coworker may offer to help you out too. But this isn't always the way things turn out. Sometimes, compassion might lead to negative results, especially if you don't learn how to use it appropriately.

CAN COMPASSION BE A WEAKNESS?

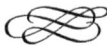

Yes, it can.

This weakness is one similarity that compassion has with empathy. Although living a compassionate life makes you a stronger and better person, you may also need to learn how to find the right balance. When you feel too much compassion, or you are always doing compassionate things for others, you might end up suffering from compassion fatigue. This is the most common situation when compassion becomes a weakness.

When you are frequently around people who need support, you may feel compassion fatigue. Naturally, this would have a powerful emotional and personal impact on your life, especially if the ones suffering are the people in your life. And when things get too much, your compassion might have adverse effects on your cognitive and emotional responses. Compassion fatigue has become so common and so detrimental that medical professionals now recognize it as an actual medical condition. So be careful when feeling compassion and taking action because of it. While it is always good to help others, this doesn't mean that you are responsible for everyone who is suffering. This is especially true if the compassion you feel is already taking a toll on your life.

It's important to learn how to take appropriate action when you feel compassion towards others. As I have said, you don't have to be the savior all the time, nor do you have to solve other people's problems for them. It's more important to show your support, give your presence, and empower others so they will be able to help themselves.

Another situation where compassion can turn into a weakness is when you allow it to quash your competitive nature. In life, we are all in competition with each other, and this doesn't have to be a negative thing. Competing with others can motivate you, make you more productive, and even make things more enjoyable for you. But when you are always worrying about how other people are doing or how they would feel if they don't come out on top, you might also be pulling yourself down. Remember, as long as you aren't hurting other people, and you aren't cheating to get where you are, compassion doesn't have to be part of the competition. If you want to help, you can try to inspire and encourage them. But you don't have to give up your drive to make others feel better as this might make you feel frustrated, resentful, or even angry in the end.

In line with this, compassion can be a negative thing when you only have it for other people. Always remember that self-compassion is just as important as feeling compassion for other people. Therefore, when you face situations where you have to choose between ending your suffering or helping ease the suffering of other people, it's okay to choose yourself. After all, how can you help others when you are suffering too?

You may have noticed how situations that make compassion a weakness only happen when compassion is

GROW WITH SYMPATHY, EMPATHY, & COMPASSION

misused or misdirected. Understanding this is the key to making sure that compassion won't end up as one of your weaknesses. When you learn how to determine whether situations call for compassion or not, then decide the most appropriate action to take, this is when you can use compassion as a tool for change. It's not that easy, but with practice, you will surely learn this as time goes by.

HOW DOES COMPASSION BECOME PAINFUL?

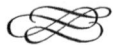

Pain is a part of life. At some point, you would experience pain from losses, injuries, heartbreaks, stresses, and more. And when you feel pain, you suffer from it. But when other people see your pain and acknowledge it, the pain seems to lessen somehow. This means that when you're on the other side of the situation —meaning you're the one who sees and acknowledges someone else's pain—you can potentially make them feel better about it.

Most people don't want to be alone when they are feeling pain, especially the emotional kind. And it's even more difficult when you are feeling pain and nobody reaches out to you, not even the ones who are physically next to you. This is where you come in with compassion. When you see someone in pain who is suffering, you can reach out and ask them about it. After hearing their story, you would feel compassion towards them; then the action comes next.

But as with empathy, when you are too compassionate, this can cause you pain too.

GROW WITH SYMPATHY, EMPATHY, & COMPASSION

When you have inner strength, you would also have the strength to show compassion. Feeling the desire to ease someone else's pain is easy, but when you realize that you cannot ease their pain, this can cause you to feel distressed. For instance, if a close friend of yours just lost someone they love, they would be in pain because of it. So you reach out, sympathize, empathize, show compassion, and start thinking about what you can do to make your friend feel better. But if your friend is in a state where they are inconsolable, try as you may, you might not be able to do anything about the pain they are feeling. Once you realize this, you might feel pained too. Even worse, the longer you stay with the person, the more painful it might be for you when all your efforts go to waste. At some point, you might even want to leave because you can't take the pain anymore. In such cases, you can either stick it out or take the easier way out and leave—just make sure that you have thought about the consequences of your decision before taking action.

In situations where compassion is causing you pain, you may want to distance yourself for a bit. Take some time off to nurture your inner self and bring back your inner strength. When the person you are showing compassion to is starting to behave in problematic or hurtful ways, it's probably best to take yourself out of that situation. Gather your thoughts and think of new ways to approach the situation. Try not to allow yourself to become a victim of physical or verbal aggression just because you feel compassion for someone else. Even if the person is your spouse or another member of your family, you don't have to allow yourself to be abused and use compassion as your excuse. Remember—self-compassion is important too, especially if you want to continue being truly compassionate towards others.

The bottom line is this: when compassion is causing you pain, you might not be using it correctly. You would feel compassion because someone is suffering, and you would do something to make things better. Your compassionate action should then make you and the other person feel better, not the other way around. Keep this in mind, and it may become easier for you to determine whether compassion is the right reaction for the situations you encounter or not.

WHEN COMPASSION DOESN'T WORK

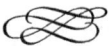

*C*ompassion doesn't come without a cost. At some point, you might feel pained, and this is what will motivate you to act. Comfort is the cost of compassion, and it is more valuable than money. When you start living with more compassion in your life, you will know what I mean by this. True compassion sometimes causes your heart to break, but you should learn and accept that you cannot help everyone. The best thing you can do is try to improve their situation to make things a little bit happier and a little less painful. And when you learn to appreciate yourself for being able to do this, your inspiration comes alive. Then you feel more motivated to keep going.

On the other hand, you would know when compassion doesn't work because it starts taking a toll on you, and it makes the situation worse. Some signs that indicate that compassion isn't working include:

- When the other person is starting to take advantage of your kindness by manipulating you into doing things for them. For instance, if

you show compassion to someone at work, and each time they are in trouble, they manipulate the situation so that you will help them out.
- When you feel guilty each time, you take action to ease the situation of the person who is suffering. For instance, if a person is in trouble with the law and you help them evade the authorities. Since you know that helping them this way is wrong, you feel guilty about it even though you know that they would suffer if they get caught.
- When the person keeps finding himself in the same dire situation because you are always there to bail them out. For instance, if you know someone who is addicted to drugs. Whenever you help the person by giving them money—which they spend on drugs—you are only enabling them to continue their addiction. Although it's painful to see the person suffer, you should change your strategy if they keep going back to the same situation.

Once you realize that compassion isn't working, it's time to change your strategy. Try to think about the situation and reflect on your reaction to it.

KNOWING WHEN THE SITUATION REQUIRES COMPASSION

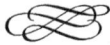

Compassion lives inside you, and all the more you practice using it, the more you learn how it works and when it is most appropriate. Acting with compassion means that you are acting from your heart. Knowing when a situation requires compassion is essential so that you can feel it, accept it, and take action that will benefit the person in need. Although compassion isn't appropriate for all kinds of situations, and some people even see it as a weakness, this doesn't mean that you should dismiss it right away.

After all, compassion isn't something you can switch off. If you feel compassion, try not to resist it. Accept it no matter what the situation it may be. But when it's time to think about the action to take, this is when you can bring in your mind to the equation. This is especially true when faced with similar situations to the ones I shared in the last section. Try to make wise decisions when it comes to the actions you take because of the compassion you feel. When you do this, it makes compassion appropriate for virtually any kind of situation.

Showing compassion toward other people also shows that you are emotionally strong. Even if you grew up in a home where those around you never showed much compassion, you could still learn it. Opening yourself up to the emotional warmth that comes from compassion allows you to experience it to the fullest. When this happens, you can allow that warmth to flow to the people around you. Take some time to feel the sense of wellbeing that comes with compassion. Even if it may feel painful at the beginning, finding ways to alleviate another person's suffering will soon turn the situation around and make things better.

The more you practice compassion (even sympathy and empathy for that matter), the more you will be able to determine when the situation requires it. Essentially, though, you will feel this with your heart. In most cases, the first time you see or hear about someone in pain, compassion is a natural response, and you don't have to resist it. But when the same situations happen to the same people over and over again, then it's time for you to start thinking about the underlying cause, as well as what you can do to help others help themselves.

True compassion is rare, and it's not that easy to master. It may take time, a conscious effort, and genuine emotion. Compassion isn't invasive, although it allows you to have direct and profound contact with the person you are feeling compassionate about. While you feel pain, you would also try to be strong so that the other person will accept the support or help you are offering. Also, compassion doesn't come with patronage or pity. It simply comes from a desire to share the vulnerability of a person in need. Through compassion, you honor the feelings of another person, accept those feelings, sometimes feel them too, and come up with a plan to turn those feelings into good ones.

As with sympathy and empathy, the moment you can

determine when a situation calls for compassion, you should use it right away. That way, you can practice compassion every time you need it until it becomes a permanent part of your life. Then, no matter what your mood is or who the person is, you will still be able to show compassion to change the lives of other people. Another thing to keep in mind when it comes to compassion is that cultivating this virtue requires a lot of self-reflection and courage. Once you accept this, compassion will come easily to you, and when faced with different kinds of situations, you will know.

PART X
USING SYMPATHY, EMPATHY, AND COMPASSION IN YOUR LIFE

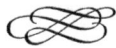

Life will always give you opportunities to use sympathy, empathy, and compassion as tools for change. No matter how dire your situation may seem at times, you will also be on the sidelines witnessing the pain and suffering of others. And when such situations happen, you should be ready for them. Throughout the chapters of this book, you have learned virtually everything you need to know about sympathy, empathy, and compassion, along with how to use them as tools of positivity. With all this information in mind, you can, hopefully, deal with different situations in positive and life-changing ways.

In this last chapter, let me share with you some scenarios where I have seen people show genuine sympathy, empathy, and compassion. These real-life scenarios will help solidify everything you have learned as you will see how these tools can promote positive changes in life—even your own.

SCENARIO 1: SHOWING SYMPATHY TO EASE THE PAIN OF LOSS

Try to imagine a scenario where I break up with my boyfriend in college. He is my high school sweetheart, the love of my life, and now that our relationship has ended, I feel shattered. I find myself walking around the neighborhood with tears streaming down my face. Lost in misery, I don't notice that my best friend is walking beside me.

She hugs me and allows me to cry. Here we are, drenched and emotional—and we stand in this powerful hug for a long time. When we finally part, she gives me a small smile and asks me if I want to talk about it. I am still in shock, but I agree to go with her to a diner. Once there, she allows me to pour my soul out. She allows me to say what I need to say, and with each word coming out of my mouth, I feel better about my situation.

Although my friend isn't do anything grand, her presence, support, and the way she doesn't judge me or try to tell me what to do make a world of difference. Once I finish talking, she comforts me with her own words and, without knowing how it happened, we are laughing about the silly things we had done in the past.

In this scenario, my friend did a superb job of showing true sympathy. My friend didn't do anything extraordinary. However, her presence, genuine support, and patience make all the difference. If you can be patient, listen well and allow people to share how they feel, you will be in a better position to offer genuine support.

SCENARIO 2: EMPATHIZING TO SHOW SUPPORT

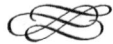

Let's try to imagine another scenario where I find out that my sister has just lost her baby before birth. To any woman, this is a truly devastating ordeal. While it may be quite easy to sympathize from afar, I can't just distance myself from the situation. After all, she is my sister, and she just experienced something extremely saddening that nobody wants to feel.

After receiving the call, my first instinct is to rush over and comfort her. But then I stop myself and take some time to reflect on the situation. I sit down, close my eyes, take a few deep breaths, and try to imagine what my sister is feeling. While I have never experienced a miscarriage before, I try to think about the emotions my sister is experiencing. This moment of self-reflection allows me to prepare myself for the moment better than I would face her unprepared.

Before going to the hospital to meet my sister, I stop by all of the places that sell her favorite comfort foods. Then the moment finally comes when I open the door to her hospital room and see her sitting there completely devastated. I hug her tight as she continues to cry. Then I tell her that I understand her feelings, and even though I have never been in the same situation, I am sharing this pain with her. Then I ask her if she needs anything to which she replies with "no." We talk for a while about what happened before moving on to other topics.

A few weeks pass, and she tells me numerous times how much I made her feel better when I told her that I shared her pain. At that time, the pain was so unbearable for her. However, the thought of having people around her who cared for her made things better, and it helped make her situation bearable.

Situations like these are not too uncommon, and you may likely have faced this type of scenario before. Because I had not experienced a miscarriage before, I didn't know how to react appropriately. Taking the time to compose myself so that I could support my sister in the best possible way was important to note. And if you ever face a situation where you are uncertain how to feel, try not to bluff your emotions. Be genuine and thoughtful—that's all anyone can ever ask from you.

SCENARIO 3: EMPATHIZING TO SPREAD HAPPINESS

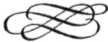

When you empathize with someone, you don't always have to share the pain, suffering, and other negative emotions. Empathy can also come into play when someone experiences something great in their life, and you share the happiness they have. One situation presented itself to me when a friend of mine received news of a promotion—her promotion was to be announced in two weeks.

Excited as my friend was, he was also a bit apprehensive. Compared to the other employees in his workplace, he was relatively new. Also, he was a lot younger than them. So, although he was excited, he also felt a bit worried about what his coworkers would think. Since I knew this friend of mine very well, it was easy for me to empathize with him. He is extremely humble and has the kindest soul. When he shared his thoughts with me, I empathized with him right away.

I knew how he felt, but I also knew that he deserved the promotion he was about to receive. I helped him realize this by telling him how much of a blessing this was to his life and how sure I was that his coworkers would be happy for him. I reminded him how much of a hard worker he was and how he was a true asset to the company. After much self-reflection and shared emotions, I had convinced him to allow himself to celebrate this good news. In this case, the empathy I felt had a positive side to it. I was proud to have helped spread happiness to my friend and his colleagues. The littlest things can upset people, and we all experience things differently. Sometimes, we need a helping hand, and if you want to grow with empathy, you should try your best to help others whenever you can.

SCENARIO 4: A CHALLENGING WAY TO SHOW COMPASSION

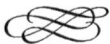

I say challenging because sometimes, we may need to get out of our comfort zones to show and appreciate genuine support. Imagine a scenario where I have been in my job for two years, and everything has been going well so far. However, during the last two weeks, my boss is quite nasty to me, doesn't give me the time to talk, and doesn't listen to my suggestions. However, this boss is generally good, and their recent behavior is quite uncharacteristic of how they normally act.

I am also going through a tough time due to my college finals, and the extra stress from my workplace is not something that I need right now. So, I tell myself that the next time that my boss is rude, I will speak up.

Of course, during my next shift, my boss snaps their fingers at me and tells me what to do and to do it quickly. At the end of my shift, before signing off, I approach my boss and ask if I can have a quick chat. They say that they only have 1 minute, and it needed to be quick.

I explain to them that their recent behavior to me has

been quite rude and inappropriate. After sharing my thoughts, the first question that I ask them is if everything okay. They bluntly reply, saying that it's none of my business, and they dismiss me.

A little confused, I leave the workplace, and a few days later, I bump into my boss at the grocery store. A little embarrassed, I hide away from him, but it's too late, and he calls out my name. I nervously walk towards him and ask how he is. He mentions that he is feeling a lot better and that he appreciates the way that I raised my concern and tried to reach out. He also mentions that he was extremely stressed because he was under pressure from his landlord.

Since the encounter, all of my shifts have been a lot more positive, and my boss seems to have things more together. To continue showing my support, now and then I ask if everything is okay with his landlord and business. He continues to thank me for being there for him.

In this scenario, after I found out that my boss was under pressure from his landlord, I decided not to tell him about my stress from my finals. Sometimes, you may need to put others in front of your needs, because it may not be so obvious why things happen the way they do. When we are compassionate, we see the good side of people more easily than when we're cloaked in negativity and judgment. However, if your boss continued to be rude, you might have to put your walls up and be a little less compassionate, so that you can have the time to take care of yourself.

One of the key themes throughout all four scenarios refers to the caring nature of genuine support that people showed to others. Sometimes, people proactively attempt to support their friends with sympathy, empathy, and compassion, such as scenarios one and two. Whereas sometimes, we only being to understand people's struggles when we start to talk with other people, such as scenarios three and four. Either way, sympathy, empathy, and compassion are powerful tools to spread happiness or support profound recovery.

Thank you for reading!

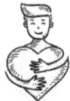 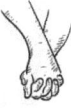 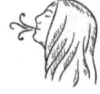 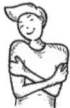

It's not over yet… there's still valuable information in the conclusion! But, if you can't wait to get your hands on unreleased chapters, sneak peeks into my next book, or free first reads of my drafts, visit the link below or scan the QR code.

kiafrost.com/earlyreader

— KIA

CONCLUSION: MAKING POSITIVE CHANGES IN YOUR LIFE

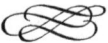

With everything you have learned about sympathy, empathy, and compassion, you can now start making positive changes in your life. Throughout this book, I've shared with practical tips and strategies along with real-life examples of sympathy, empathy, and compassion in action that I hope you find helpful.

With everything you have learned here, the one thing that I want you to take away from this book is a choice to become a better person. Living a more compassionate life balanced with just the right amounts of sympathy and empathy will make you a beacon of hope to others. And the best part is, you don't even have to force yourself into doing difficult things. As long as you apply the simple tips I have shared, sympathy, empathy, and compassion will come more naturally to you. And when you can gain some mastery of using these tools, you will see how much they can improve the lives of those around you.

Naturally, when you can help other people out, this will make you feel better. Trust me; when you see the light in another person's eyes because you gave them something that other people are struggling with or you can help them in ways other people never thought of using, you will understand why sympathy, empathy, and compassion are considered as powerful, life-changing tools.

I wish you well on your journey towards a more positive, enlightened, and mindful life filled with love, happiness, and genuine connections with others.

ABOUT THE AUTHOR

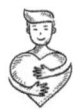 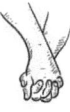 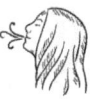 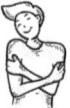

Kiannah Frost is the author of "Grow with Sympathy, Empathy, & Compassion." Kia focuses on providing high-quality writing that is easy to read and simple to understand. She aims to help her readers translate words into actions so that they can apply their knowledge in the real world.

Kia describes herself as a full-time learner of all things related to Psychology. She has an academic background in Psychology and experience in research with a specialty in human behavior.

If you have been searching for ways to help other people out in more profound ways, Kia recommends her first release titled "Grow with Sympathy, Empathy, & Compassion."

REFERENCES

3 Inspiring Ways to Show Sympathy. (2016). Retrieved from https://www.spoonfulofcomfort.com/blog/3-inspiring-ways-to-show-sympathy/

Abrugar, V. Q. (n.d.). 20 Ways to Show Compassion to Others. Retrieved from https://inspiringtips.com/ways-to-show-compassion-to-others/

Armstrong, K. (n.d.). 'I Feel Your Pain': The Neuroscience of Empathy. Retrieved from https://www.psychologicalscience.org/observer/i-feel-your-pain-the-neuroscience-of-empathy

Babauta, L. (n.d.). zenhabits : breathe. Retrieved from https://zenhabits.net/a-guide-to-cultivating-compassion-in-your-life-with-7-practices/

Bariso, J. (2016). The 1 Lesson That Will Sharpen Your Emotional Intelligence. Retrieved from https://www.inc.com/justin-bariso/emotional-intelligence-101-the-difference-between-sympathy-and-empathy.html

Barnes, E. L. (2017). What Empathy Is Not. Retrieved from https://dotdev.co/what-empathy-is-not/

Beard, M. (2014). The world is burning, but remember

REFERENCES

our sympathy goes only so far | Matthew Beard. Retrieved from https://www.theguardian.com/commentisfree/2014/jul/22/the-world-is-burning-but-remember-our-sympathy-goes-only-so-far

Becker-Phelps, L. (2018). Can You Be Too Compassionate? Retrieved from https://www.psychologytoday.com/au/blog/making-change/201801/can-you-be-too-compassionate

Ben-Zeév, A. (2010). Do Not Pity Me. Retrieved from https://www.psychologytoday.com/us/blog/in-the-name-love/201008/do-not-pity-me

Benefits of Empathy. (n.d.). Retrieved from http://cultureofempathy.com/References/Benefits/

Brown , S., Brown , R. M., & Preston, S. (2011). The Human Caregiving SystemA Neuroscience Model of Compassionate Motivation and Behavior. Retrieved from https://www.researchgate.net/publication/279722795_The_Human_Caregiving_SystemA_Neuroscience_Model_of_Compassionate_Motivation_and_Behavior

Bariso, J. (2016, April 21). The 1 Lesson That Will Sharpen Your Emotional Intelligence. Retrieved from https://www.inc.com/justin-bariso/emotional-intelligence-101-the-difference-between-sympathy-and-empathy.html

Burton, N. (2015). Empathy vs. Sympathy. Retrieved from https://www.psychologytoday.com/au/blog/hide-and-seek/201505/empathy-vs-sympathy

Burton, N. (2015). Empathy vs. Sympathy. Retrieved from https://www.psychologytoday.com/au/blog/hide-and-seek/201505/empathy-vs-sympathy

Chernyak, P. (2019). How to Express Sympathy. Retrieved from https://www.wikihow.com/Express-Sympathy

REFERENCES

Cherry, K. (2019). Why Is It Important to Use Empathy in Certain Situations? Retrieved from https://www.verywellmind.com/what-is-empathy-2795562

Chua, C. (2019). 8 Tips to Be Empathetic to Others. Retrieved from https://personalexcellence.co/blog/empathy

Cohen, E. D. (2015). How to Be Empathetic. Retrieved from https://www.psychologytoday.com/au/blog/what-would-aristotle-do/201505/how-be-empathetic

Compassion. (n.d.). Retrieved from https://www.skillsyouneed.com/ps/compassion.html

Compassion. (2020). Retrieved from https://en.wikipedia.org/wiki/Compassion

Compassion Definition: What Is Compassion? (n.d.). Retrieved from https://greatergood.berkeley.edu/topic/compassion/definition

Dibakar, P. (2011). Of Sympathy. Retrieved from https://papers.ssrn.com/sol3/papers.cfm?abstract_id=1763305

Dodgson, L. (2018). Having too much empathy can lead us to burn out - but there are ways to use it as a superpower. Retrieved from https://www.businessinsider.com/how-not-to-burn-out-from-empathy-2018-6

Empathy vs. Sympathy. (2019). Retrieved from https://www.grammarly.com/blog/empathy-sympathy/

Empathy vs. Sympathy: Which Word To Use And When. (2019). Retrieved from https://www.dictionary.com/e/empathy-vs-sympathy/

Endersby, S. (2018). What are the advantages of sympathy? Retrieved from https://www.quora.com/What-are-the-advantages-of-sympathy

Ewers, P. (2017). 5 Actionable Tips to Develop Empathy and Become a More Empathetic Person.

REFERENCES

Retrieved from https://mindmaven.com/blog/5-tips-to-become-more-empathetic/

Firestone, R. W. (2013). How to Stop Playing the Victim Game. Retrieved from https://www.psychologytoday.com/us/blog/the-human-experience/201304/how-stop-playing-the-victim-game

Galang, K. M., Schraps, P., & Rigby, T. (2019). Why is sympathy important? Retrieved from https://www.quora.com/Why-is-sympathy-important

Gilbert, P. (2013). How to Turn Your Brain from Anger to Compassion. Retrieved from https://greatergood.berkeley.edu/article/item/how_to_turn_brain_anger_compassion

Gillihan, S. J. (2016). Presence, Pain and Compassion. Retrieved from https://www.psychologytoday.com/us/blog/think-act-be/201601/presence-pain-and-compassion

Goins, J. (2011). The Cost of Compassion: Why It Feels Bad to Do Good. Retrieved from https://goinswriter.com/cost-of-compassion/

Gu, X., Gao, Z., Wang, X., Liu, X., Knight, R. T., Hof, P. R., & Fan, J. (2012). Anterior insular cortex is necessary for empathetic pain perception. Retrieved from https://www.ncbi.nlm.nih.gov/pubmed/22961548

Harley, M. (2018). The Benefits Of Compassion & Self Compassion. Retrieved from https://lifelabs.psychologies.co.uk/users/3881-maxine-harley/posts/30673-the-benefits-of-compassion-self-compassion

Holland, K. (2018). How to Recognize the Signs of Emotional Manipulation and What to Do. Retrieved from https://www.healthline.com/health/mental-health/emotional-manipulation

Hougaard, R., & Carter, J. (2018). The Dangers of

Being an Empathetic Leader. Retrieved from https://www.entrepreneur.com/article/311413

How to be happy: Compassion is a strength, not a weakness. (2011). Retrieved from https://www.independent.co.uk/life-style/health-and-families/healthy-living/how-to-be-happy-compassion-is-a-strength-not-a-weakness-5334365.html

How To Express Sympathy: What To Say And What Not to Say. (n.d.). Retrieved from https://www.everplans.com/articles/how-to-express-sympathy-what-to-say-and-what-not-to-say

Illing, S. (2019). The case against empathy. Retrieved from https://www.vox.com/conversations/2017/1/19/14266230/empathy-morality-ethics-psychology-compassion-paul-bloom

Jankowiak-Siuda, K., Rymarczyk, K., & Grabowska, A. (2011). How we empathize with others: a neurobiological perspective. Retrieved from https://www.ncbi.nlm.nih.gov/pmc/articles/PMC3524680/

Jazaieri, H. (2018). Six Habits of Highly Compassionate People. Retrieved from https://greatergood.berkeley.edu/article/item/six_habits_of_highly_compassionate_people

Krawczyk, K. (2018). 10 Ways to Show Compassion. Retrieved from https://montessorirocks.org/10-ways-to-show-compassion/

Krznaric, R. (2012). Six Habits of Highly Empathic People. Retrieved from https://greatergood.berkeley.edu/article/item/six_habits_of_highly_empathic_people1

Lasaki, F. (2017). When Empathy Goes Wrong. Retrieved from https://thriveglobal.com/stories/when-empathy-goes-wrong/

Levy, R., & Diedrich, R. A. (2018). Why do people often consider compassion as a weakness? Retrieved from

REFERENCES

https://www.quora.com/Why-do-people-often-consider-compassion-as-a-weakness

Lonczak, H. (2019). 20 Reasons Why Compassion Is So Important in Psychology. Retrieved from https://positivepsychology.com/why-is-compassion-important/

Malti, T., Gummerum, M., Keller, M., & Buchmann, M. (2009). Children's moral motivation, sympathy, and prosocial behavior. Retrieved from https://www.ncbi.nlm.nih.gov/pubmed/19467003

Mamas, M. (2016). Keys to Being Compassionate - The Strength of Vulnerability. Retrieved from https://medium.com/@michaelmamas/keys-to-being-compassionate-the-strength-of-vulnerability-90adf312e189

Markham, L. (2013). When Empathy Doesn't "Work". Retrieved from https://www.psychologytoday.com/us/blog/peaceful-parents-happy-kids/201307/when-empathy-doesnt-work

Mazie, S. (2014). Five Reasons You Should Be Less Empathetic. Retrieved from https://bigthink.com/praxis/five-reasons-you-should-be-less-empathetic

McManus, M. R. (2020). How Empathy Works. Retrieved from https://science.howstuffworks.com/life/inside-the-mind/emotions/empathy.htm

Miller, C. C. (n.d.). How to Be More Empathetic. Retrieved from https://www.nytimes.com/guides/year-of-living-better/how-to-be-more-empathetic

Mochel, D. (2017). If Compassion Is a Weakness, Then I Want to Be As Weak As Possible. Retrieved from https://www.huffpost.com/entry/if-compassion-is-a-weakness-then-i-want-to-be-as-weak-as-possible_b_8723416

Molenberghs, P. (2019). Understanding others' feelings: what is empathy and why do we need it? Retrieved from https://theconversation.com/understanding-others-feelings-what-is-empathy-and-why-do-we-need-it-68494

REFERENCES

Neilson, E. (n.d.). The Do's and Don'ts of Expressing Sympathy. Retrieved from https://tomorrow.me/trustworthy/life-skills/the-dos-and-donts-of-expressing-sympathy/

Orloff, J. (2017). The Science Behind Empathy and Empaths. Retrieved from https://www.psychologytoday.com/us/blog/the-empaths-survival-guide/201703/the-science-behind-empathy-and-empaths

Park, N., Peterson, C., Szvarca, D., Vander Molen, R. J., Kim, E. S., &Collon, K. (2014). Positive Psychology and Physical Health: Research and Applications. Retrieved from https://www.ncbi.nlm.nih.gov/pmc/articles/PMC6124958/

Rajmohan, V., & Mohandas, E. (2007). Mirror neuron system. Retrieved from https://www.ncbi.nlm.nih.gov/pmc/articles/PMC2900004/

Rand, D. G., Greene, J. D., & Nowak, M. A. (2012). Spontaneous giving and calculated greed. Retrieved from https://www.nature.com/articles/nature11467

Riess, H. (2017). The Science of Empathy. Retrieved from https://www.ncbi.nlm.nih.gov/pmc/articles/PMC5513638/

Roy, S. (2020). 5 Dangers Of Empathy: How Empathy Hurts. Retrieved from https://happyproject.in/empathy-hurts/

Rube, T. (2020). How to Show Empathy. Retrieved from https://www.wikihow.com/Show-Empathy

Schairer, S. (2017). What's the Difference Between Empathy, Sympathy, and Compassion? Retrieved from https://chopra.com/articles/whats-the-difference-between-empathy-sympathy-and-compassion

Schwarz, R. (2013). What Stops Leaders from Showing Compassion. Retrieved from https://hbr.org/2013/08/what-stops-leaders-from-showin

REFERENCES

Segal, E. A. (2018). Five Ways Empathy Is Good for Your Health. Retrieved from https://www.psychologytoday.com/us/blog/social-empathy/201812/five-ways-empathy-is-good-your-health

Seltzer, L. F. (2014). The Downside of Compassion. Retrieved from https://www.psychologytoday.com/us/blog/evolution-the-self/201403/the-downside-compassion

Seppala, E. (n.d.). The Compassionate Mind. Retrieved from https://www.psychologicalscience.org/observer/the-compassionate-mind

Seppala, E. (2013). Compassionate Mind, Healthy Body. Retrieved from https://greatergood.berkeley.edu/article/item/compassionate_mind_healthy_body

Stern, R., &Divecha, D. (2015). How to Avoid the Empathy Trap. Retrieved from https://greatergood.berkeley.edu/article/item/how_to_avoid_the_empathy_trap

Sympathy. (2019). Retrieved from https://en.wikipedia.org/wiki/Sympathy

Sympathy and Condolence Advice. (2019). Retrieved from http://www.legacy.com/news/advice-and-support/article/sympathy-and-condolence-advice

Sympathy vs. Empathy vs. Compassion. (n.d.). Retrieved from http://operationmeditation.com/discover/sympathy-vs-empathy-vs-compassion/

Sympathy vs. Empathy: What's the Difference? (n.d.). Retrieved from https://www.merriam-webster.com/words-at-play/sympathy-empathy-difference

Sympathy, Empathy, Compassion, and Pity - How Are They the Same and How Are They Different? (2019). Retrieved from https://riseservicesinc.org/sympathy-empathy-compassion-pity/

The Advantage Of Sympathy. (2016). Retrieved from https://bluetoadpublishing.co.uk/publication/?m=

REFERENCES

18570&i=296911&view=articleBrowser&article_id=2451523&ver=html5

The Psychology of Emotional and Cognitive Empathy. (n.d.). Retrieved from https://lesley.edu/article/the-psychology-of-emotional-and-cognitive-empathy

Tremaine, L. (2018). 9 Powerful Benefits of Compassion. Retrieved from https://leightremaine.com/9-powerful-benefits-of-compassion/

Types of Empathy. (n.d.). Retrieved from https://www.skillsyouneed.com/ips/empathy-types.html

Understanding the Meaning of Compassion. (n.d.). Retrieved from https://www.compassion.com/child-development/meaning-of-compassion/

UnderwoodMay, E. (2015). Rats forsake chocolate to save a drowning companion. Retrieved from https://www.sciencemag.org/news/2015/05/rats-forsake-chocolate-save-drowning-companion

Vermeiren, J. (2018). Sympathy, Empathy and Compassion. Retrieved from https://www.thecompassionateleader.org/sympathy-empathy-and-compassion/

Warneken, F., Hare, B., Melis, A. P., Hanus, D., &Tomasello, M. (2007). Spontaneous altruism by chimpanzees and young children. Retrieved from https://www.ncbi.nlm.nih.gov/pmc/articles/PMC1896184/

Ways to Show Sympathy: Condolences Examples. (n.d.). Retrieved from https://www.dignitymemorial.com/support-friends-and-family/ways-to-show-sympathy

Welsh, I. (2018). The Problem With Empathy and the Advantage of Sympathy. Retrieved from https://www.ianwelsh.net/the-problem-with-empathy-and-the-advantage-of-sympathy/

What is Compassion? And How Can I Be More

REFERENCES

Compassionate? (2018). Retrieved from https://www.compassionuk.org/blogs/what-is-compassion/

What is Sympathy? (n.d.). Retrieved from https://www.skillsyouneed.com/ips/sympathy.html

What to Do When Compassion Doesn't Work. (2017). Retrieved from https://susangaddis.net/2014/08/when-compassion-does-not-work/

Williams, J. A. (n.d.). What Is Empathy and Why Is It Important? Retrieved from https://blog.heartmanity.com/what-is-empathy-and-why-is-it-important

Winder, A. (2019). 5 Benefits of Empathy (and How to be More Empathetic). Retrieved from https://goals.com/5-benefits-of-empathy-and-how-to-be-more-empathetic

www.ingramcontent.com/pod-product-compliance
Lightning Source LLC
Chambersburg PA
CBHW070043230426
43661CB00005B/733